SURGERY – PROCEDURES, COMPLICATIONS, AND RESULTS SERIES

HAND SURGERY: PREOPERATIVE EXPECTATIONS, TECHNIQUES AND RESULTS

SURGERY – PROCEDURES, COMPLICATIONS, AND RESULTS SERIES

Hand Surgery: Preoperative Expectations, Techniques and Results
Robert H. Beckingsworth (Editor)
2010. ISBN: 978-1-60876-280-4

Surgery – Procedures, Complications, and Results Series

Hand Surgery: Preoperative Expectations, Techniques and Results

Robert H. Beckingsworth
Editor

Nova Biomedical Books
New York

For permission to use material from this book please contact us:
Telephone 631-231-7269; Fax 631-231-8175
Web Site: http://www.novapublishers.com

Library of Congress Cataloging-in-Publication Data

Hand surgery : preoperative expectations, techniques and results / editor, Robert H. Beckingsworth.

p. ; cm.

Includes bibliographical references and index.

ISBN 978-1-60876-280-4 (hardcover : alk. paper)

1. Hand--Surgery. 2. Hand--Wounds and injuries. I. Beckingsworth, Robert H.

[DNLM: 1. Hand--surgery. 2. Hand Injuries--surgery. 3. Tissue Engineering--methods. WE 830 H2334 2009]

RD559.H3599385 2009

617.5'75059--dc22 2009031118

Published by Nova Science Publishers, Inc. ✈ New York

Contents

Preface

The field of hand surgery deals with both surgical and non-surgical treatment of conditions and problems that may take place in the hand or upper extremity (commonly from the tip of the hand to the shoulder). Hand surgery may be practiced by graduates of general surgery, orthopedic surgery and plastic surgery. Plastic surgeons are particularly well suited to handle traumatic hand and digit amputations that require a "replant" operation. Hand surgeons perform a wide variety of operations such as fracture repairs, releases, transfer and repairs of tendons and reconstruction of injuries, rheumatoid deformities and congenital defects. This new and important book gathers the latest research from around the globe in the study of hand surgery and focuses on such topics as: stem cell applications in hand surgery, tissue engineering for bone repair in the hand, intramedullary fixation of distal radius fractures and others.

Chapter 1 - Tissue is frequently damaged or lost in injury and disease. There has been an increasing interest in stem cell applications and tissue engineering approaches in surgical practice to deal with damaged or lost tissue. Tissue engineering is an exciting strategy being explored to deal with damaged or lost tissue. It is the science of generating tissue using molecular and cellular techniques, combined with material engineering principles, to replace tissue. This could be in the form of cells with or without matrices. Although there have been developments in almost all surgical disciplines, the greatest advances are being made in orthopaedics, especially in cartilage repair. This is due to many factors including the familiarity with bone marrow derived mesenchymal stem cells and cartilage being a relatively simpler tissue to engineer. Unfortunately significant hurdles remain to be overcome in many areas before tissue engineering becomes more routinely used in clinical practice.

Cells used in tissue engineering could be autologous, allogeneic or xenogeneic. The cells could be stem cells or cells further down the differentiation pathway. The use of embryonic stem cells is associated with religious, political and social concerns, but the use of adult stem cells is generally well accepted. Stem cells have been identified in a number of adult tissues, albeit in small numbers. In addition to bone marrow, mesenchymal stem cells have been identified in a number of tissues including adipose tissue and fat pad. The mesenchymal stem cells are generally isolated from the tissue and expanded in culture. These cells are characterised or defined using a set of cell surface markers; mesenchymal stem cells are generally positive for CD44, CD90 and CD105, and are negative for haematopoetic markers

CD34 and CD45, and the neurogenic marker CD56. These cells can be differentiated down a particular differentiation pathway e.g. osteoblast or chondrocyte, using predefined culture conditions before being used for clinical applications. In this chapter stem cells are discussed in detail followed by the tissue engineering approaches for articular cartilage.

Chapter 2 - Injuries and disease commonly affect the hand and these can significantly affect the ability of an individual to perform activities of daily living. The use of regional outcome measures or scoring systems is important as it allows comparison between these injuries and disease, and allows clinicians to assess progression and the effects of different treatment modalities. A patient-completed questionnaire is efficient in terms of time and resources, and allows the assessment of outcome without the need to attend an outpatient clinic.

It is important that the scoring system allows satisfactory regional outcome measurements specific for the hand. This is particularly important in injuries and disease that involve both upper and lower limbs. The validity, reliability, responsiveness and bias are used for the assessment of various questionnaires. The validity establishes whether the outcome measure actually measures what it was designed to. The criterion, construct, and content or face validity provide various assessment parameters that allow a complete picture of the validity of a questionnaire to be established. An outcome tool has test-retest reproducibility if the same result is obtained when tested at different time points once the condition has stabilised. The responsiveness is the ability to detect clinically important changes in disability at various intervals. The effect size and the standardised response mean are used to evaluate the responsiveness. Bias can occur when assumed independent variables such as age, gender, hand dominance or dominant side injured affect responses. There are also many practical issues concerning the use of questionnaires including feasibility of use for the patient and the clinician.

The Disability of the Arm, Shoulder and Hand (DASH) questionnaire, the Patient Evaluation Measure (PEM) questionnaire, and the Michigan Hand Outcome (MHO) questionnaire are a few of the region-specific outcome measures commonly used for the hand, and are patient-completed questionnaires. They are frequently used to assess self-reported patient outcome in orthopaedics, rheumatology and neurology. In this chapter, the validity, reliability, responsiveness and bias of the various questionnaires used for the assessment of the hand will be discussed.

Chapter 3 - Tissue is frequently damaged or lost in injury and disease. There has been an increasing interest in stem cell applications and tissue engineering approaches in surgical practice to deal with damaged or lost tissue. Tissue engineering is an exciting strategy being explored to deal with damaged or lost tissue. It is the science of generating tissue using molecular and cellular techniques, combined with material engineering principles, to replace tissue. This could be in the form of cells with or without matrices. Although there have been developments in almost all surgical disciplines, the greatest advances are being made in orthopaedics, primarily because of familiarity with bone marrow derived mesenchymal stem cells and experience with using materials for scaffolds. Unfortunately significant hurdles remain to be overcome in many areas before tissue engineering becomes more routinely used in clinical practice. In this chapter the tissue engineering approaches relevant to hand surgery for tendons, skin, nerves and blood vessels will be discussed.

Chapter 4 - Tissue is frequently damaged or lost in injury and disease. There has been an increasing interest in stem cell applications and tissue engineering approaches in surgical practice to deal with damaged or lost tissue. Tissue engineering is an exciting strategy being explored to deal with damaged or lost tissue. It is the science of generating tissue using molecular and cellular techniques, combined with material engineering principles, to replace tissue. This could be in the form of cells with or without matrices. Although there have been developments in almost all surgical disciplines, the greatest advances are being made in orthopaedics, especially in bone repair. This is due to many factors including the familiarity with bone marrow derived mesenchymal stem cells and bone grafting. Unfortunately significant hurdles remain to be overcome in many areas before tissue engineering becomes more routinely used in clinical practice. In this chapter the tissue engineering approaches relevant to hand surgery for bone repair will be discussed. Significant hurdles however remain to be overcome before tissue engineering becomes more routinely used in surgical practice.

Chapter 5 - Arthrodesis of the wrist has been considered as the gold standard for osteoarthritis of the wrist. In 1984 Watson and Ballet (1) recognized a specific pattern of carpal collaps (SNAC), other alternatives have been proposed: the proximal row carpectomy (PRC) and the scaphoidectomy combined with a four corner arthrodesis. In this cohort of 54 patients, two motion preserving procedures were compared (26 PRC's and 28 four corner fusions)

The PRC had significantly better outcome for range of motion and DASH. Grippping force was not significantly different between both procedures

Chapter 6 - Pain in the area of the ulnar wrist remains a diagnostic and therapeutic challenge for the hand surgeon. Better delineation of the possible etiologies of ulnar wrist pain and correlation with their clinical, arthroscopic, and radiographic findings is critical to enhancing our ability to treat these patients. The authors suggest a primary distinction between intraarticular pathology (in the ulnocarpal joint) and extraarticular pathology. This organization provides the basis for the algorithmic approach presented in this chapter.

Intraarticular causes include TFCC tears, ulnar impaction, and lunotriquetral tears Extraarticular causes encompass ulnar styloid triquetral impaction, ulnar impingement, DRUJ arthritis, pisotriquetral joint dysfunction, hamate and triquetral fractures, and ECU disorders. A novel extraarticular cause of ulnar-sided wrist pain, Triquetral Impingement Ligament Tear (TILT) syndrome, is presented. Each of these causes has specific symptoms and findings on physical and radiographic exam. Arthroscopy is useful for diagnosis and treatment of intraarticular problems, and can confirm isolated extraarticular disease when intraarticular findings are normal. The algorithm presented in this chapter aids the clinician in making the correct diagnosis and choosing the appropriate treatment.

Chapter 7 – Introduction: Distal radius fracture alignment and stabilization can be a surgical challenge in the face of severe comminution and bone loss. The current standard of care for such cases calls for autologous bone grafting and rigid fixation. In this chapter, we describe a technique using HydroSet (Stryker), a calcium phosphate bone cement, as an adjunct to internal fixation. The technique eliminates the need for autologous bone grafting and the associated donor site morbidity. This bone graft substitute is biocompatible, osteoconductive, and sets quickly with an isothermic reaction. Available bone cements, studies involving the use of bone cement for distal radius fractures, indications, and surgical technique will be reviewed.

Methods: All consecutive severely comminuted distal radius fractures treated by the senior author over a period of 9 months using standard surgical technique and rigid fixation were reviewed. Six females and seven males with an average age of 50.7 (+/-15.9) met criteria. HydroSet bone cement was used in 14 fractures in 14 patients. Radiographs were used to assess healing.

Results: Bony healing was achieved in all but one patient. Severe dorsal comminution with loss of articular surface and articular support was present in 9 cases. In all of these cases HydroSet was used to reconstruct the dorsal articular surface. In one case, the HydroSet was used to reconstruct over 80% of the articular surface. Screws were not drilled into the HydroSet. No collapse was seen on radiographs at 6 weeks follow-up.

Discussion: Bioactive bone cements hold great promise for the treatment of comminuted distal radius fractures. In our case series the use of bone cement eliminated the need for primary autologous bone grafting. It allowed for easier reduction and retention of reduction at the time of surgery due to the quick hardening time. The graft did not allow for screw insertion, and therefore the hardware was used as a buttress for the graft. As there usually was no cavity bound on three sides by bone, post-operative X-rays are full of visible bone graft and are difficult to interpret. However, radial length was maintained 6 weeks postoperatively. Despite limited follow up, the clinical results using HydroSet bone cement are encouraging.

Chapter 8 - The goal of internal fixation of the distal radius fracture is restoration of the disrupted anatomy and early return to function while minimizing soft tissue trauma and prolonged immobilization. This has been achieved with standard plating techniques, particularly volar locked-plates. More recently, intramedullary fixation has experienced increased interest as an alternate option for distal radius fracture fixation. Intramedullary fixation permits limited soft tissue dissection and insertion of a low profile that acts as an internal splint. The use of intramedullary fixation for displaced distal radius fractures utilizes the accepted principles of stable fracture fixation and early motion but also provides the additional benefits of load-sharing and decreased soft tissue irritation. Purported benefits include a familiar fracture fixation technique, less soft tissue irritation, and locked fixed-angle technology.

Thorough understanding of the radial and dorsal approaches to the distal radius is a prerequisite. Surgical technique involves (1) fracture reduction, (2) nail insertion, and (3) locking screw placement. Important aspects of intramedullary fixation of distal radius fractures include proper fracture selection, good fracture reduction, protection of sensory nerves, and avoidance of inadvertent intra-articular screw placement. Fractures indicated for intramedullary fixation include predominantly displaced extra-articular or simple intra-articular distal radius fractures.

Chapter 9 - Implants used in the hand and wrist have to satisfy certain criteria. They should be small, biomechanically strong enough to withstand loading in the hand and wrist and should have a low profile. In addition to these features, it is extremely useful, if they are inert enough to avoid causing local soft tissue or bony reaction and therefore do not require additional procedures for removal. Bioabsorbable implants fulfill all these criteria, and although their use in the hand and wrist is still in its infancy, early data suggest that the rates of success and complications associated with their use, are comparable to that associated with their metal counterparts. As costs associated with their production and use reduce, and more data regarding their efficacy become available, it appears that universal acceptance will follow.

In: Hand Surgery: Preoperative Expectations... ISBN: 978-1-60876-280-4
Editor: Robert H. Beckingsworth

Chapter 1

Stem Cell Applications and Cartilage Tissue Engineering Approaches Applicable in Hand Surgery

Wasim S Khan[1*] ***and Timothy E Hardingham***[2]
[1]University College London Institute of Orthopaedics and Musculoskeletal Sciences, Royal National Orthopaedic Hospital, Stanmore, London, HA7 4LP, UK
[2]UK Centre for Tissue Engineering and Wellcome Trust Centre for Cell Matrix Research, Faculty of Life Sciences, University of Manchester, Manchester, M13 9PT, UK

Abstract

Tissue is frequently damaged or lost in injury and disease. There has been an increasing interest in stem cell applications and tissue engineering approaches in surgical practice to deal with damaged or lost tissue. Tissue engineering is an exciting strategy being explored to deal with damaged or lost tissue. It is the science of generating tissue using molecular and cellular techniques, combined with material engineering principles, to replace tissue. This could be in the form of cells with or without matrices. Although there have been developments in almost all surgical disciplines, the greatest advances are being made in orthopaedics, especially in cartilage repair. This is due to many factors including the familiarity with bone marrow derived mesenchymal stem cells and cartilage being a relatively simpler tissue to engineer. Unfortunately significant hurdles remain to be overcome in many areas before tissue engineering becomes more routinely used in clinical practice.

Cells used in tissue engineering could be autologous, allogeneic or xenogeneic. The cells could be stem cells or cells further down the differentiation pathway. The use of

* Corresponding Author: Mr Wasim S Khan, Academic Clinical Fellow, University College London Institute of Orthopaedics and Musculoskeletal Science, Royal National Orthopaedic Hospital, Stanmore, London, HA7 4LP, UK Telephone number: +44 (0) 7791 025554 Fax number: +44 (0) 20 8570 3864 E-mail address: wasimkhan@doctors.org.uk

embryonic stem cells is associated with religious, political and social concerns, but the use of adult stem cells is generally well accepted. Stem cells have been identified in a number of adult tissues, albeit in small numbers. In addition to bone marrow, mesenchymal stem cells have been identified in a number of tissues including adipose tissue and fat pad. The mesenchymal stem cells are generally isolated from the tissue and expanded in culture. These cells are characterised or defined using a set of cell surface markers; mesenchymal stem cells are generally positive for CD44, CD90 and CD105, and are negative for haematopoetic markers CD34 and CD45, and the neurogenic marker CD56. These cells can be differentiated down a particular differentiation pathway e.g. osteoblast or chondrocyte, using predefined culture conditions before being used for clinical applications. In this chapter stem cells are discussed in detail followed by the tissue engineering approaches for articular cartilage.

Introduction

Orthopaedic surgery in general and hand surgery in particular has been highly successful in repairing, realigning and replacing damaged musculoskeletal structures. The coming years will establish whether a paradigm shift from fixation towards regeneration of tissue is possible, clinically feasible and financially viable. In developing tissue engineering techniques based on mesenchymal stem cells, a better understanding of these cells, their various sources, their characterisation and their differentiation potential will be crucial in devising personalised treatment strategies suited to individual patients and lesions. Without this knowledge, there is a risk that suboptimal cell-based treatments will fare misleadingly badly in comparative clinical studies.

Stem Cells

Stem cells are a self-renewing, slow-cycling cell population that exhibit high clonogenity, low cellular proliferation and the ability to undergo multilineage differentiation. Humans originate from the ultimate stem cell, the fertilised egg, and develop through a process of cell proliferation and differentiation. The cell undergoes several early divisions producing more totipotent cells, blastomeres that give rise to the embryonic membranes, placenta and the embryo. The self-renewing property of the stem cell is manifest by either symmetric or asymmetric cell divisions; symmetric divisions result in in the propagation of two stem cells or the production of two terminally differentiated cells, whereas asymmetric cell division results in one stem cell and one terminally differentiated cell. The cells have a hierachy of differentiation potential with the cells at the top of the heirachy derived from the first few cell divisions after fertilisation. Further down are the embryonic stem cells derived from the inner cell mass of the blastocyst. These pluripotent cells can differentiate into any of the three germ layers of ectoderm, mesoderm and endoderm. During embryonic development, stem cells from the blastocyst give rise to cell progenies that become progressively restricted in their phenotypic potential to generate mature tissue. At advanced stages of development, the product of stem cells may be a multipotent cell with limited degree of differentiation, lower self-renewal potential, and a higher cell proliferation rate. Adult somatic cells are usually terminally differentiated or have restricted phenotypes they can adopt under specific culture conditions. The cell divisions eventually produce terninally differentiated cells that are unable to renew and eventually undergo apoptosis (Alison et al, 2002; Triffitt, 2002). Many adult tissues maintain populations of cells that are not terminally differentiated. These postnatal stem cells are required for normal tissue remodelling and repair. They can be isolated from tissues of individuals of any age and maintain some capacity for multilineage differentiation.

Embryonic Stem Cells

The culture of embryonic stem cells derived from the blastocyst was first described by Thomson et al in 1998. These cells have generated considerable interest as a potential source for tissue engineering because of their high telomerase activity allowing them to proliferate indefinitely *in vitro,* and maintainence of their pleuripotency (de Wert and Mummery, 2003; Vats et al, 2005). Donor embryonic stem cells will however need to be histocompatibility leucocyte antigen (HLA)-matched to the recipient as a prerequeset to clinical application. Transplanted embryonic stem cells have caused teratomas in mouse models highlighting the need for using only fully differentiated cells in the clinical setting (Orkin and Morrison, 2002). These findings, as well as the potential in higher passage cells of epigenic and genetic changes resulting in an abnormal karyotype with trysin or collagenase IV (Draper et al, 2004), raise serious safety issues.

Adult Mesenchymal Stem Cells

Experiments performed by Friedenstein and co-workers described the presence of mesenchymal stem cells (MSCs) in the bone marrow (Friedenstein 1966; Friedenstein 1968). Friedenstein demonstrated that these cells could be isolated through their intrinsic property to adhere to tissue culture plastic (Friedenstein 1970). These cells formed colonies of cells with spindle-like fibroblastic appearance *in vitro*, and they were initially termed colony forming unit-fibroblasts (CFU-Fs). *In vitro* studies have shown that CFU-Fs are a heterogeneous population of stem cells at different levels of heirachy (Owen et al, 1987; Owen and Friedenstein, 1988). MSCs are cells derived from the mesoderm and are defined as cells that can give rise to a variety of mesenchyme derived cell types including chondrocytes, osteoblasts, adipocytes, myoblasts and hepatocytes (Prockop, 1997; Pittenger et al, 1999). These cells have considerable therapeutic potential for the repair and regeneration of tissue. By the end of last century, there was considerable interest in the use of MSCs for clinical tissue engineering applications highlighted by the work of Pittinger et al (1999) showing that cells could differentiate *in vitro* into the three mesenchymal lineages of chondrocytes, osteoblasts and adipocytes.

Stem cells possess self-renewal capacity, and exhibit long-term viability and multilineage differentiation potential. Ethical, political and religious issues surround the use of embryonic stem cells. In contrast, the use of autologous postnatal MSCs is generally well accepted by society. MSCs are less tumourogenic than their embryonic counterparts (Raghuath et al, 2005) and provide an autologous source of cells eliminating concerns regarding rejection and disease transmission. There is also evidence to suggest that MSCs have immunosuppressive potential as co-culture with MSCs inhibits T-cell lymphocyte proliferation (Krampera et al, 2003), and MSCs have also been shown to be negative for major histocompatability complex (MHC) class II antigens and the co-stimulatory molecules B7-1 and B7-2 (Devine and Hoffman, 2002; Majumdar et al, 2003) and they are being tested in clinical trials to treat GVHD (graft-versus-host-disease) arising from bone marrow allografts (Le Blanc et al, 2004) and also for the treatment of Crohn's disease (inflammatory bowel disease) and COPD (chronic obstructive pulmonary disease). All these factors support the use of MSCs for the creation of a more marketable off-the-shelf tissue engineered product.

Sources of Adult Mesenchymal Stem Cells

Cells with stem cell characteristics have been isolated from many different adult tissues including cord blood, peripheral blood, bone marrow, spleen, liver, kidney, thymus, dental pulp, periosteum, skin, retina, adipose tissue, skeletal muscle, synovial tissue and the synovial infrapatellar fat pad (Johnstone et al, 1998; Erices et al, 2000; De Bari et al, 2001; Zuk et al, 2001; Dragoo et al, 2003; Peng and Huard, 2003; Wickham et al, 2003). The choice of stem cell source is determined by ease of access to tissue source, frequency of stem cells and information on a particular cell system. More recent published work also suggests that MSCs from different tissues vary in their differentiation potential (Zuk et al, 2002; Sakaguchi et al, 2005).

Bone Marrow Derived Mesenchymal Stem Cells

Bone marrow derived stem cells have been widely studied and there is a wealth of information in literature concerning them. Adult mammalian bone marrow contains two discrete stem cell populations, haematopoietic stem cells and MSCs (Pittinger et al, 1999; Short et al, 2003). Protocols for the culture (Freidenstein et al, 1970) and, chondrogenic, osteogenic and adipogenic differentiation of bone marrow derived MSCs have been described (Johnstone et al, 1998; Pittenger et al, 1999; Sekiya et al, 2002). However not all stromal cells derived from bone marrow are MSCs. These cells form only 0.001-0.01% of the total nucleated cells in bone marrow aspirates (Jones et al, 2002). Harvesting of bone marrow is painful with donor site morbidity and risk of wound infection and sepsis (Pittenger et al, 1999). Bone marrow aspirate of 30 ml only produces approximately $1x10^5$ cells (Bruder et al, 1997a) making expansion in culture necessary. Obtaining a large number of cells at harvest has the potential advantage of not needing costly and time-consuming tissue culture expansion that risks cell contamination.

Synovial Fat Pad Derived Stem Cells

The synovial infrapatellar fat pad or Hoffa's fat pad is an intracapsular but extrasynovial structure. It lies on the inferior aspect of the patella behind the patellar ligament and in front of the synovial lined knee joint (William et al, 1989). It is a flexible and displaceable structure. The volume varies and it is lost only in extreme emaciation after subcutaneous fat is eliminated (Saddik et al, 2004). The fat pad is similar in structure to subcutaneous adipose tissue containing fibrous tissue interspersed among adipose tissue. It may contain horizontal and vertical synovial lined clefts that communicate with the synovial cavity (Smillie et al, 1974; LaPrade, 1998). The synovial fat pad has a rich blood supply that is derived from an anastamosis of vertically orientated vessels from the superior and inferior genicular arteries. These vertical vessels are then further interconnected by horizontal vessels (Kohn et al, 1995; Kim et al, 1996).

MSCs extracted from synovial fat pad have been induced into chondrogenic, adipogenic and osteogenic phenotype using appropriate media (Dragoo et al, 2003; Wickham et al, 2003). Some papers describe the synovial fat pad as adipose synovium (Mochizuki et al, 2006), since the synovium covers the fat pad and the subsynovium comprises of adipose connective tissue. These cells have been shown to have a cell surface molecule profile similar but not identical to that of bone marrow derived MSCs, and maintain their multipotency into the later stages of life (Wickham et al, 2003).

Compared to bone marrow, synovial fat pad is reported to give a higher yield of adherent colony forming cells; bone marrow aspirate of 30 ml produced approximately 1 x 10^5 cells (Bruder et al, 1997a), whereas 21 ml of synovial fat pad yielded approximately 5.5 x 10^6 cells (Dragoo et al, 2003). There is reduced pain and morbidity associated with the harvest of synovial fat pad cells compared with bone marrow cells (Dragoo et al, 2003). In a patient matched quantitative comparison looking at MSCs from five sources, synovial tissue derived cells showed better proliferation and chondrogenic potential under the conditions tested compared to cells from bone marrow, adipose tissue, periosteum and skeletal muscle (Sakaguchi et al, 2005). They also showed better osteogenic potential, along with bone marrow and periosteum derived cells, and better adipogenic potential along with adipose tissue derived stem cells. In another study, fat pad derived cells were shown to be more similar in their cell surface epitope profile, and proliferative, chondrogenic and osteogenic differentiation potential to synovial tissue derived cells than to adipose tissue derived cells (Mochizuki et al, 2006).

Synovial fat pad derived MSCs are a possible alternative to differentiated chondrocytes in autologous chondrocyte implantation for the repair of focal cartilage defects. Compared to cells harvested from the bone marrow, these cells are easier to obtain, have lower donor site morbidity and are associated with a higher yield of MSCs (Dragoo et al, 2003). A biopsy from these tissues may represent an easily accessible source of mesenchymal stem cells at diagnostic or therapeutic arthroscopy. The synovial fat pad is commonly resected at arthroscopy and total knee arthroplasty for improved surgical visualisation, and in arthroplasty to prevent possible impingement of the fat by the prosthesis. No adverse long-term side effects have been noted following the resection of the synovial fat pad (Duri et al, 1996). It is also resected for chronic impingement and fibrosis of the fat pad (Hoffa's disease)

(Ogilvie-Harris and Giddens, 1994). To enable their use in cell-based repair strategies, it is crucial that more is known about the exact nature of these cells.

Age-Related Changes in Mesenchymal Stem Cells

The reported effects of ageing on MSCs are variable. A number of studies have shown an age-related decline in the number and proliferation of bone marrow derived MSCs (D'Ippolito et al, 1999; Shamsul et al, 2004; Bertram et al, 2005; Huang et al, 2005b; Mareschi et al, 2006; Stolzing et al, 2008; Zhou et al, 2008), however a number of other studies found no difference (Stenderup et al, 2001; Suva et al, 2004; Scharstuhl et al, 2007). Our preliminary experiments on bone marrow derived MSCs showed no significant age-related changes in cell proliferation and characterisation supporting the work of Mareschi et al (2006). A number of studies have shown an age-related change in the differentiation potential of bone marrow derived MSCs (Jiang et al, 2008; Zhou et al, 2008), but this has not been reported in some other studies (Stenderup et al, 2001; Huang et al, 2005b; Roura et al, 2006; Scharstuhl et al, 2007; Siddappa et al, 2007). Scipper et al (2008) compared adipose tissue derived MSCs and noted differences in cell proliferation and PPAR-gamma-2 expression related to age. The applicants have previously looked at the effects of ageing in later life (age 50-90 years) on the isolation, expansion, cell surface characterisation and osteogenic potential of synovial fat pad derived MSCs and found no difference (Khan et al, in press). Much of the conflicting data in the literature may be due to variations between patients and in the culture conditions used. In this proposed study, the effect of such variations will be reduced via examinations of the effect of age on the phenotype, proliferation and differentiation potential of patient-matched samples during identical culture conditions.

A potential cell source that does not show age-related decline in proliferation and differentiation is important in determining the optimal cell-based tissue repair therapies in an aging population. An ideal source of stem cells would be easy to obtain with a small risk of complications, with a good cell yield not requiring long culture expansion and exhibit good proliferation and differentiation potential.

Differentiation of Stem Cells

MSCs have been shown to differentiate into chondrocytes, osteoblasts and adipocytes under appropriate culture conditions (Pittenger et al, 1999). Predifferentiation of MSCs will be essential in clinical applications to ensure appropriate lineage commitment and to avoid undesired tissue formation and heterotopic tissue formation. The presence of only the *in vivo* environment alone is not sufficient to allow chondrogenesis (Wakitani et al, 1994; Manne et al, 2005). Chondrogenesis has been shown to occur in MSCs cultured as cell aggregates with specific differentiation and growth factors (Johnstone et al, 1998; Mackay et al, 1998). Chondrogenic differentiation of such cells requires specific medium with TGF β and a three-dimensional culture environment e.g. as a cell aggregate, to allow differentiation *in vitro*.

This shows that cell density, contact and topography also contribute to the process (Johnstone et al, 1998; Pittenger et al, 1999; Sekiya et al, 2002). Mackay et al (1998) showed that high glucose medium and TGF β3 are needed for the chondrogenic differentiation of MSCs. Insulin-like growth factor-1 (IGF1) has been shown to have a synergistic effect with TGF β in promoting chondrogenesis in MSCs (Indrawattana et al, 2004). The end point is the accumulation of cartilage matrix gene products as demonstrated by gene expression and immunostaining of collagen types II, IX and XI, and aggrecan.

Chondrocyte differentiation can be divided into three stages: cell condensation, chondrocyte differentiation and chondrocyte hypertrophic maturation. TGF β has a role in cell condensation, probably by inducing the expression of Sry-related HMG box-9 (SOX9) (Furumatsu et al, 2005). SOX9 regulates the expression of aggrecan and collagen types II, IX and XI during chondrocyte differentiation (Magne et al, 2005a). SOX5 and SOX6 are also expressed early during chondrocyte differentiation, but their exact molecular mechanisms remain uncertain (Akiyama et al, 2002). Hypoxia inducible transcription factor-1 (HIF1) makes chondrocyte survival possible in hypoxic conditions (Schipani et al, 2001). Hypertrophic differentiation is characterized by the expression of collagen type X.

Adipogenic and osteogenic differentiation can also be demonstrated with the same cell population (Pittenger et al, 1999), but the detailed molecular mechanisms driving differentiation into these different cell phenotypes have not yet been elucidated. Monolayer culture of mesenchymal stem cells with standard osteogenic medium containing β-glycerophosphate, dexamethasone and ascorbate have been shown to induce osteogenic differentiation (Beresford et al, 1994). Adipogenesis in undifferentiated MSCs is comprised of two stages: determination of the adipocyte lineage and adipogenic differentiation. The molecular pathways involved in the second stage have been studied extensively (Gregoire, 2001) but those for the first stage are not well understood (MacDougald & Mandrup, 2002). It has previously been reported that the adipogenic differentiation of MSCs is only possible when the cells are confluent (Ishino et al, 2004). MSCs require several cycles of hormonal stimulation to exit from the cell cycle: a feature necessary to achieve commitment to the adipogenic lineage (Ramirez-Zacarias et al, 1992).

Insulin, dexamethasone and 3-isobutyl-1-methyl xanthine (IBMX) have been shown to be sufficient to stimulate adipogenic differentiation (Pittinger et al, 1999; Zuk et al, 2001; Rim et al, 2005). Insulin is needed to generate the substrate glycerol 3-phosphate, which is needed for the biosynthesis of triglycerides (Sottile & Seuwen, 2001). Insulin is known to promote the proliferation and differentiation of pre-adipocytes (Ailhaud, 1982). High concentrations of insulin mimic the role of IGF1 (Qiu et al, 2001) and have a mitogenic effect. The anti-inflammatory drug indomethacin is a peroxisome proliferator-activated receptor gamma-2 (PPARγ2) activator and is a strong inducer of adipogenesis (Rosen & Spiegelman, 2000).

Optimisaton of Chondrogenic Differentiation Potential

Stem cells are defined by their self-renewal and multipotentiality. Unfortunately these crucial properties appear to show considerable donor variability and become limited on expansion in monolayer culture as these cells lose their proliferation and differentiation potential (Pittinger et al, 2001; Cancedda et al, 2003). As expansion in culture is needed to increase the cell number to a level suitable for clinical applications, it is important to explore avenues that would allow for this expansion without a significant compromise of differentiation potential.

Cells are normally cultured *in vitro* in an atmosphere of 5% carbon dioxide in standard tissue culture incubators. As the remaining gas consists of air, oxygen levels are almost 20% (140 mm Hg). It has long been known that some cells, including some with stem cell characteristics, proliferate more rapidly in lower oxygen concentrations (Rich and Kubanek, 1982; Rich, 1986). These cells include human periosteal cells (Deren et al, 1990), haematopoietic progenitor cells (Koller et al, 1992) and neural crest stem cells (Morrison et al, 2000). This would appear feasible since the partial pressure in arterial blood is 75-110 mm Hg and that in bone marrow is 27-49 mm Hg (Lennon et al, 2001). Culture in low oxygen selectively enhances collagen type II expression and cartilage matrix assembly (Adesida et al, 2006), and appears to be a major and selective control at the translational level with upregulation of collagen processing enzymes.

Articular cartilage is avascular and exists at reduced oxygen tension of 1-7% in vivo depending on the depth from the articular surface (Silver, 1975; Wang et al, 2005). So, it is not surprising that hypoxia is also known to increase the synthesis of extracellular matrix components of chondrocytes (Murphy and Sambanis, 2001; Domm et al, 2002). In stem cells derived from bone marrow (Scherer et al, 2004), adipose tissue (Wang et al, 2005) and synovial fat pad (Khan et al, 2007), hypoxia has also been shown to improve chondrogenesis.

Monolayer expansion is associated with a flattened cell morphology in stem cells and in primary chondrocytes. Chondrocytes have been shown to maintain their chondrogenic phenotype when cultured under conditions that prevent cell flattening e.g. high-density cell aggregate culture (Watt, 1988) or three-dimensional scaffolds, and by supplementation of actin disrupting agents (Loty et al, 1995). FGF-2 has been shown to induce disassembly of the actin microfilament architecture (Wroblewski and Edwall-Arvidsson, 1995). Disruption of actin microfilaments results in the upregulation of SOX9 mRNA (Tew & Hardingham, 2006), and this may be the pathway involved in maintaining the chondrogenic phenotype.

FGF-2 is also a potent mitogen for a variety of cell types derived from the mesoderm including chondrocytes (Kato & Gospodarowicz, 1985). The potential of passaged articular chondrocytes to be chondrogenic has been shown to be enhanced by rapid expansion with a medium containing PDGF-BB, TGF β3 and FGF-2 (Hardingham et al, 2002; Martin et al, 2003; Li et al 2004). FGF-2 has been shown to enhance proliferation and differentiation of bone marrow (Martin et al, 1997; Bianchi et al, 2003; Solchaga et al, 2005) and synovial fat pad (Khan et al, 2008) derived MSCs. FGF also has a role in *in vivo* cartilage repair when released from bone matrix where it is stored, and following local exogenous administration into osteochondral defect cavities (Hiraki et al, 2001).

Stem Cell Markers

Most cell surface markers are inadequate in identifying stem cells unambiguously either because these markers are also expressed by non-stem cells, or they are only expressed by stem cells at a particular stage and under particular culture conditions (Pittinger & Martin, 2004). Tables 1 and 2 shows known cell markers for bone marrow derived haematopoietic stem cells and MSCs, and synovial fat pad derived MSCs. Bone marrow MSCs are uniformly positive for CD29, CD44, CD71, CD90, CD105 and CD106, and are negative for markers of haematopoetic lineage including CD14, CD34 and CD45 (Haynesworth et al, 1992; Barry et al, 1999; Pittenger et al, 1999; Jones et al, 2002). Chondrogenic potential appears to be related to the expression of CD105, a TGF β receptor, recognised by SH2 (Barry et al, 1999; Ragunath et al, 2005).

Table 1. Cell markers used in the characterization of mesenchymal stem cells and their characteristics.

Cell Marker	Characteristics
3G5	Monoclonal antibody that recognises CD44v3
STRO-1	Murine IgM monoclonal antibody that identifies a trypsin insensitive unidentified cell surface antigen on bone marrow derived MSCs
αSMA	Alpha smooth muscle actin, specific for smooth muscle fibres
αLNGFR	Receptor for low affinity nerve growth factor
SH2	Monoclonal antibody that identifies CD105
SH3	Antibody that identifies CD73
SH4	Antibody that identifies CD73
SB-10	Monoclonal antibody that recognises CD166
CD10	Common acute lymphocytic leukaemia antigen
CD11b	Integrin αM subunit
CD13	Aminopeptidase N
CD14	Component of lipopolysaccharide receptor on lymphocytes
CD29	Integrin β1 subunit
CD34	Cell surface glycoprotein of haematopoietic lineage
CD44	Receptor for hyaluronan
CD44v3	Receptor for a ganglioside on pericytes in the vasculature
CD45	Leucocyte common antigen, a protein tyrosine phosphatase
CD49a	Integrin alpha subunit
CD56	Neural cell adhesion molecule (NCAM)
CD73	GPI-linked cell surface protein involved in B cell activation
CD90	GPI-linked cell surface protein Thy-1
CD105	Endoglin; TGF β receptor type III
CD106	Vascular cell adhesion molecule 1 (VCAM-1)
CD146	MCAM/Muc-18, antigen on endothelail cells
CD166	ALCAM, Type I membrane glycoprotein adhesion molecule on activated leucocytes
D7FIB	Marker of human fibroblast/epithelial cells
vWF	von Willebrand factor: product of endothelial cells/platelets

Table 2. Cell markers for bone marrow derived haematopoietic stem cells and MSCs in aspirate and culture, and for synovial fat pad derived MSCs.

Tissue	Cell markers
Bone marrow derived haematopoietic stem cells	CD14, CD34, CD45 (Haynesworth et al, 1992) CD11b, CD34, CD45 (Baddoo et al, 2003)
Bone marrow derived MSCs in aspirate	αSMA (Shi & Granthos, 2003) αLNGFR (Quirici et al, 2002) STRO1, CD106 (Simmons & Torok Stork, 1991; Dennis et al, 2002; Shi & Gronthos, 2003) LNGFR, STRO1, CD10, CD13, CD90, CD105 (Jones et al, 2002)
Bone marrow derived MSCs in culture	CD29, 44, 106 (Baddoo et al, 2003) αSMA (Shi & Granthos, 2003) SH2, SH3, SH4, CD44, CD90 (Pittenger et al, 1999) SH2, SH3, SH4 (Haynesworth et al, 1992)
Synovial fat pad derived MSCs	CD13, CD29, CD44, CD59, CD105 (Wickham et al, 2003) CD 44, CD90, CD105, CD147 (Mochizuki et al, 2006)

Bone marrow derived MSCs are selected from fresh aspirate as STRO1 and CD106 positive (Dennis et al, 2002; Shi & Gronthos et al, 2003). CD34 contains many cell types in addition to early progenitor and stem cells, and STRO1 antibody was developed to differentiate MSCs from other CD34 positive cells in the bone marrow (Simmons & Torok Stork, 1991; Gronthos et al, 1994; Gronthos et al, 1999). STRO1 does not bind to haematopoietic progenitor cells but binds to bone marrow derived MSCs (Dennis & Caplan, 2000; Dennis et al, 2002). It identifies an as yet uncharacterised cell surface molecule.

Alpha smooth muscle actin (αSMA) is also expressed by freshly isolated bone marrow derived MSCs and 70% of the STRO1 positive cells express αSMA (Shi and Gronthos, 2003). Monoclonal antibodies to the alpha low affinity nerve growth factor receptor (αLNGFR) stain freshly isolated bone marrow MSCs but do not label haematopoietic cells (Quirici et al, 2002). Baddoo et al (2003) used a combination of plastic adherence and in vitro culture along with the removal of contaminating haematopoietic cells by negative selection using antibodies to CD11b, CD34 and CD45. The resulting cells were shown to express CD29, CD44 and CD106. This describes phenotypical properties of bone marrow MSCs based on analysis of marrow stromal cells in culture. Jones et al (2002) reported these cells to be uniformly positive for LNGFR, STRO1, CD10, CD13, CD90 and CD105, and negative for CD14, CD34, CD117 and CD133.

Wickham et al (2003) showed that more than 50% of the synovial fat pad derived cells in culture were positive for CD13, CD29, CD44, CD59 and CD105. Mochizuki et al (2006) showed that the same proportion of cells were positive for CD44, CD90, CD105 and CD147. Other potential MSC markers for culture-expanded MSCs include CD10, CD31, CD49a, CD54, CD55, CD73, CD146 and CD166 (Vaananen, 2005). Antibody SB-10 reacts with CD166 (Bruder et al, 1998a) and SH3 and SH4 identify CD73 (Barry et al, 2001). We have shown that all bone marrow derived MSCs (unpublished data) and fat pad derived MSCs (Khan et al, 2007) stain strongly for CD13, CD29, CD44, CD90 and CD105.

A full characterisation of synovial fat pad derived MSCs is important to achieve a greater understanding of their origin and their repair potential. *Ex vivo* expanded cells may need to undergo a large number of cell divisions in monolayer culture to reach a number sufficient for clinical applications. It has previously been reported that MSCs retain their pleuripotency for 6-10 passages (Spees et al, 2004). De Bari et al (2001) showed that the cell surface epitope profile of synovial tissue derived MSCs was stable during expansion from passage 3 up to at least passage 10. We have shown that the cell surface characterisation of mesenchymal stem cells derived from the synovial fat pad is maintained with expansion in FGF-2 (Khan et al, 2008), with ageing in later life and (Khan et al, 2009) and with expansion up to passage 18 (unpublished data).

Problems with Stem Cell Markers

There is a lack of specific cell markers for selectively isolating stem cells. There are also potential problems with the use of cell surface markers including some variability in expression dependant on culture conditions (Bruder et al, 1997b; Stewart et al, 1999; Quirici et al, 2002).

STRO1 cross-reacts with erythroblasts. CD10, CD13 and CD90 are expressed on human fibroblasts as well as bone marrow derived MSCs (Jones et al, 2002). CD105 is also expressed on endothelial cells and early B lineage precursor cells in bone marrow (Barry et al, 1999; Deans and Moseley, 2000). CD44 and CD29 have broad cell reactivity (Jones et al, 2002; Quirici et al, 2002). Although CD34 is a haematopoetic stem cell marker, it is also expressed by endothelial cells (Miranville et al, 2004). Some studies report the expression of CD34 in MSCs isolated from the bone marrow, though they state that it is rapidly lost after in vitro culture (Quirici et al, 2002). The expressions for STRO-1 (Bruder et al, 1997b; Stewart et al, 1999) and LNGFR (Quirici et al, 2002) are also progressively lost in culture. This may be because of the progressive loss in culture of non-proliferating cells or presence of high proportions of foetal calf serum in the culture medium inhibiting the expression of some surface antigens (Garcia-Pacheco et al, 2001).

The use of a large number of markers and the negative selection procedures are used to deal with this problem. Pittinger et al (1999) reported the use of several antibodies to characterise expanded MSC populations from bone marrow.

Pericytes as Candidate Stem Cells

It has been suggested that bone marrow derived MSCs originate from microvascular pericytes (Bianco et al, 2001; Short et al, 2003). The exact nature and location of stem cells in the synovial fat pad, or indeed any tissue, is not known.

The inner layer comprising of a single layer of longitudinally arranged flattened epithelial cells is called the endothelium. This is supported by a basement membrane, collagenous tissue and an internal elastic lamina in arteries. This together with endothelium forms the tunica intima. The tunica media is the intermediate muscular layer and contains circumferentially arranged vascular smooth muscle cells. The tunica adventitia is the outer supporting tissue layer that merges with the surrounding collagenous tissue and may contain the external elastic lamina. Fibroblasts are the predominant cell type in this layer.

In arteries the amount of elastic tissue decreases with size and there is an increase of the smooth muscle content. Arterioles are vessels with a lumen of less than 0.3 mm in diameter. They have a thin internal elastic lamina and no external elastic lamina. The tunica media is composed of smooth muscle cells in six concentric layers or less. The tunica adventitia may be as thick as the tunica media. In venules, the elastic and muscular components are much less prominent. A characteristic feature is the wide lumen diameter relative to the wall thickness. Muscular venules have an intimal layer with no elastic fibres and a medial layer consisting of one or two layers of smooth muscle fibres. Capillaries consist of a single layer of flattened endothelial cells lining the capillary lumen. Muscular and adventitial layers are absent. Pericytes in the form of flattened cells embrace the endothelial cells.

The term 'pericyte' originates from its early anatomical descriptions ('peri-' around and 'cyto-' cell) reflecting its periendothelial location of these cells. Pericytes are cells closely associated with capillaries and were first described by Rouget in 1873 (Hirschi and D'Amore, 1996). Vascular pericytes are cells that were initially characterised as associated with retinal capillaries. The embryonic origin of pericytes remains unknown but it is suggested that they may be derived from the mesenchyme (Nayak et al, 1988). They are embedded within a basement membrane and are separated from the endothelial cells, that they surround, by the basal lamina that allows interdigitation (Nayak et al, 1988). They cover microvasculature arterioles, capillaries and venules on their abluminal surface. Pericytes are thought to be a heterogeneous cell population exhibiting tissue-related and vessel-related characteristics (Hirshi and D'Amore, 1996). Within the blood vessel, pericytes have a contractile function and are thought to control local blood flow (Hirschi and D'Amore, 1996). They also play an important role in microvessel stability, structural integrity, vasodynamic capacity, permeability and control of angioneogenesis (Hirschi and D'Amore, 1997; Thomas, 1999).

The cell biology of pericytes was largely developed by investigation of retinal peicytes isolated from bovine eyes and these were of particular interest as potential sources of vascular calcification. Pericytes isolated from bovine retinal capillaries were reported to be STRO1 positive (Doherty et al, 1998) and exhibited potential for differentiation into a variety of cell types including osteoblasts (Brighton et al, 1992), smooth muscle cells (Meyrick et al, 1981), adipocytes and chondrocytes (Rhodin, 1968; Farrington-Rock et al, 2004). Pericytes have also been reported in other tissues such as dental pulp as antibody 3G5 positive cells (Bankfalvi et al, 1998; Nayak et al, 1988), and in bone marrow as STRO1 positive cells (Doherty et al, 1998; Shi and Gronthos, 2003). Pericytes, like bone marrow MSCs, express STRO1, αLNGFR and αSMA in culture (Herman and D'Amore, 1985; Wesseling et al, 1995; Jones et al, 2004).

αSMA is also expressed by freshly isolated bone marrow MSCs *in vitro*, and 70% of the STRO1 positive cells express αSMA (Shi and Granthos, 2003). αSMA has restricted distribution in bone marrow *in vivo* in the vascular smooth muscle cells in the tunica media of the arteries and pericytes, and occasional flattened cells on the endosteal surface of bone (Bianco et al, 2001).

The periosteal pericytes are in the correct anatomical location for migration into the bone marrow during development. It has been suggested that if distributed more widely with capillaries, pericytes could account for stem cells in other tissues (Gronthos et al, 2003). In support of this theory, a continuous subendothelial network of pericyte like cells has been identified using 3G5 throughout the entire human vascular bed (Andreeva et al, 1998). Indeed, many of the tissues from which stem cells have been isolated have good vascularisation. A minor population of bone marrow derived MSCs has been found to be positive for the cell surface ganglioside recognised by antibody 3G5 (Shi & Gronthos, 2003).

Articular Cartilage

Articular or hyaline cartilage is a specialised connective tissue that is avascular, aneural and alymphatic. It is a load bearing tissue supported by underlying subchondral bone. Chondrocytes are the only cell type and there is a low cell turnover. These cells are highly specialised cells that secrete the extracellular matrix proteins. They function by maintaining the integrity of the cartilage by balanced synthetic and catabolic activities. The extracellular matrix is composed of a complex combination of predominantly type II and lesser amounts of type VI, IX and XI collagen fibrils specifically arranged with large water retaining aggrecan molecules and other smaller proteoglycans bonded to them. This combination gives cartilage the ability to resist repetitive compressive load bearing without premature wear (Poole, 1995; Hardingham, 1998).

Collagens contain a unique triple-helical peptide structure with a repeating motif, with glycine as every third amino acid and a high frequency of proline. These molecules are arranged in fibrils with overlapping and cross-linking of adjacent molecules. The main collagen in cartilage is collagen type II forming 80-90% of the total content. It is a long chain fibrillar collagen that forms the major fibre network of the tissue. Collagen type XI is also a long chain fibrillar collagen and accounts for almost 3% of the total collagen content in cartilage. Collagen type IX is found on the outside of type II fibrils, and has a special structure possibly to allow interactions with other fibrils and proteoglycans. Collagen type VI may have a role in cell-matrix interactions. Collagen type X is a short chain collagen that occurs specifically in calcifying cartilage produced by hypertrophic chondrocytes in the growth plate (Hardingham, 1998).

The interfibrillar matrix is filled with proteoglycan. The main proteoglycan in cartilage is aggrecan that consists of a large core protein with polysaccharide chains attached to it including chondroitin sulphate and keratan sulphate. At the N-terminal of the protein core there are two globular domains G1 and G2. The G1 domain acts as a site for aggregation of aggrecan molecules, and allows binding to hyaluronan and link protein (Hardingham, 1998). Almost 70% of the cartilage wet weight is water and this contributes to the load-bearing properties of the tissue. The glycosoaminoglycan (GAG) chains attached to proteoglycans carry a high density of negative charge. This attracts positively charged ions and creates an osmotic pressure that draws water into the tissue (Hardingham & Fosang, 1992).

Embryology

Articulating joints start forming embryologically within cartilage long bone rudiments with the appearance of regions of high cell density, interzones, where cells lose the expression of chondrocyte-specific markers such as collagen type II. These cells differentiate and form three layers. The central layer has a lower cell density and the cells die through apoptosis creating a joint cavity. Cells on either side differentiate to form articular chondrocytes. Adult articular cartilage can also be divided into three layers. The surface zone is characterised by flattened, discoid cells that mainly secrete proteoglycan. The mid zone contains rounded cells arranged in columns that mainly secrete collagen type II and aggrecan. The deeper zone is calcified and contains collagen type X (Eyre, 1991; Magne et al, 2005).

Growth Plate Cartilage

Bone is formed through two separate developmental processes where mesenchymal cells are recruited into condensations before differentiation on receiving signals elicited by factors such as members of the transforming growth factor beta (TGFβ) superfamily. In intramembranous ossification, the cells directly commit to become osteoblasts, but in endochondral ossification, the cells first form a cartilaginous template in the form of the growth plate. The cells in the centre of the condensations differentiate into chondrocytes promoted by strong SOX9 activation and low Wnt/β-catenin signalling. Later in development, the growth plate chondrocytes become flattened and organised into columns. These chondrocytes express early markers such as collagen type II, IX and XI, and aggrecan. The cells on the peripheries of the condensation form the perichondrium and differentiate into osteoblasts.

The chondrocytes then further differentiate to become prehypertrophic chondrocytes and then hypertrophic chondrocytes that express collagen type X and calcify their extracellular matrix. The hypertrophic maturation of the chondrocytes is under the control of the Ihh/PTHrP loop; Ihh expressed in prehypertrophic cells induces the expression of PTHrP in the cells located in the perichondrium. PTHrP in turn inhibits hypertrophic differentiation and failure of its signalling results in Blomstrand chondroplasia. Members of the Wnt family on the other hand trigger hypertrophic differentiation. These hypertrophic chondrocytes eventually die through apoptosis and the vascular invasion of the calcified cartilage brings osteoclasts and osteoblasts (Karsenty and Wagner, 2002; Magne et al, 2005).

Osteoarthritis

Articular cartilage is frequently damaged by trauma and in joint disease, such as osteoarthritis but shows only a limited capacity for repair. This is due to the lack of inherent mechanisms of repair in mature articular cartilage. Cartilage defects that extend to the subchondral bone show some signs of repair with the formation of neocartilage (Newman,

1998) probably due to the release of bone marrow derived stem cells from the underlying subchondral bone (Shapiro et al, 1993).

Osteoarthritis is the most prevalent disorder of the musculoskeletal system. Approximately fifteen percent of the total UK population suffers from arthritis, and seventy percent of the population over the age of 65 years will limit their activities or seek medical attention because of osteoarthritis. It has a significant impact on the ability to perform the activities of daily living (Simon, 1999). This together with the increasing age of the population and the costs involved in management of this disorder make it a major social issue, especially in industrialised developed countries with high life expectancy (Buckwalter, 2002). A total knee or hip replacement costs the National Health Service (NHS) between four and eight thousand pounds and the additional cost to the individual in terms of socio-economic consequences with loss of earnings and productively, and social and psychological upset is significantly higher. This is the driving force behind numerous ongoing efforts to develop new tissue-engineered strategies for the treatment of osteoarthritis (Schulz and Bader, 2007).

Pathophysiology of Osteoarthritis

The main pathological features of osteoarthritis, including cartilage failure, are characterised by dysregulation of tissue turnover in articular cartilage and subchondral bone. This leads to an imbalance between dynamic reparative and catabolic processes (Hardingham, 1998), where both increased cartilage matrix turnover and increased production are inviolved. The tissue damage may be driven by local production of inflammatory cytokines e.g. tissue necrosis factor alpha (TNF α) and interleukin-1 beta (IL-1β) and protease release by cells in cartilage, synovium and bone (Risbud and Sittinger, 2002) and the anabolic response in cartilage may involve local release of FGF2 (Chia et al, 2009), but may also be contributed to by TGFβs, bone morphogenic proteins (BMPs) and insulin-like growth factor-1 (IGF1). This leads to a loss of proteoglycan and disruption of the collagenous fibrillar network. While osteochondral defects show some evidence of attempts at repair with the formation of neocartilage (Newman, 1998), chondral defects do not. This is probably due to the release of bone marrow derived stem cells and growth factors in cartilage defects that extend to the underlying subchondral bone (Shapiro et al, 1993; Newman, 1998).

The patients frequently complain of pain, stiffness and swelling of the joints that leads to reduced exercise tolerance and poorer quality of life. The first line of management is a trial of non-operative treatment that includes analgesia or anti-inflammatory medication, physiotherapy and occupational therapy. The articular cartilage shows only a limited capacity for repair and current treatments are aimed at relieving inflammation and pain and do little to delay disease progression (Wollheim, 1996; Simon, 1999).

Current Surgical Treatment Modalities

Most patients with osteoarthritis end up requiring surgical intervention. A few options for the repair of focal cartilage lesions have been used in larger joints including abrasive chondroplasty, subchondral drilling, microfracture and cartilage transplantation. In subchondral drilling and microfracture, bone marrow derived stem cells are stimulated to migrate from the subchondral bone to the site of cartilage defect. This however results in the formation of fibrocartilage rather than hyaline cartilage. Histologically, fibrocartilage contains more fibrous tissue, and biochemically contains significantly less proteoglycan and more collagen type I. Fibrocartilage has inferior mechanical and hydroelastic characteristics and results in unsatisfactory clinical outcome (Hunziker, 2001). Cartilage transplantation is limited by donor availability and is only available in a few centres with variable results (O'Driscoll, 1998; Bentley and Minas, 2000; Hunziker, 2001). Most focal cartilage lesions, left untreated, progress to more extensive lesions and these require extensive surgical procedures in the form of joint arthroplasty or arthrodesis.

The frequent outcome when pain and loss of function become severe is surgical intervention for joint replacement or arthrodesis. Joint replacement is successful for elderly patients, but the limited lifetime of prostheses makes it much less desirable for younger patients. Younger patients are more likely to return to a more active lifestyle putting increased stresses and strains on their joint replacement (Parsons and Sonnabend, 2004). This means a greater likelihood of needing a revision procedure with its associated increased operative complications.

Autologous Chondrocyte Implantation

For joint problems in younger patients there is great interest in the potential of cell-based strategies to provide a biological repair of cartilage. Autologous chondrocytes are being used for the repair of focal cartilage defects in larger joints combined with a periosteal or resorbable collagen membrane sutured to the cartilage surface (Brittberg et al, 1994, 2001, 2003). These principles could also apply as proof-of-principle to focal defects in the hand. Although this technique was initially described for the knee, it has now been extended to the hip, ankle, shoulder, elbow and wrist joint (Brittberg et al, 2003). This is becoming a generally accepted technique for the repair of focal defects in the articular cartilage and has proved superior to mosaicoplasty in a prospective controlled clinical trial (Bentley et al, 2003). The first stage of the procedure entails an initial biopsy from a low weight bearing part of the articular cartilage. This is digested and mature articular chondrocytes are retrieved. These are then expanded in monolayer culture *ex vivo* for three weeks. The proliferation allows the number of chondrocytes to increase. Chondrogenesis is confirmed by gene expression for collagen type II and aggrecan, and histochemical and biochemical analysis. The cells are then trypsinised and ready for reimplantation at the second stage. The second stage involves an arthrotomy, debridement of articular defect and suturing of a periosteal or resorbable collagen membrane sealed with fibrin glue. The cells are then delivered under the membrane and the wound is closed. The cells settle, adhere, proliferate and lay down new cartilage (Brittberg et al, 2003).

The procedure has demonstrated usefulness, but would benefit from further development. It is a two-step procedure, it is expensive and technique-dependant. The procedure involves cartilage biopsy from the joint to obtain the chondrocytes and the periosteum, which therefore involves injury to the low weight bearing cartilage surface at initial biopsy and possible injury to the periosteum at the second procedure with associated morbidity of the donor site. It has only limited applications i.e. for focal cartilage defects, in view of the amount of tissue that can be obtained. Human articular chondrocytes are not easily extractable. The small amount of tissue also means that cell expansion in culture is necessary, and this is generally slow (Homicz et al, 2002). With prolonged expansion chondrocytes lose their ability to proliferate (Risbud and Sittinger, 2002; Cancedda et al, 2003) and their ability to express cartilage specific proteins (Benya & Shaffer, 1982). Also, the number of cell divisions these cells can undergo reduces with age and deteriorating health restricting the expansion potential of these cells (Dozin et al, 2002). These cells, when implanted, result in the formation of fibrocartilage rather than the desired hyaline cartilage (Clar et al, 2005). Although short-term clinical results have been good, evidence suggests progression of degenerative changes in the joint (Lee et al, 2000a).

The current autologous chondrocyte procedure thus implants cells with variable chondrogenic potential. It is thus less than ideal to use autologous chondrocytes harvested from the same joint.

Tissue Engineering Approaches for Articular Cartilage Defects

Articular cartilage is a particularly suitable tissue for tissue engineering applications as it is avascular, aneural and alymphatic. Articular cartilage shows a limited capacity for repair following injury. Cartilage injuries that extend down to the subchondral bone show some signs of repair due to the release of bone marrow derived mesenchymal stem cells from the subchondral bone, a principle used in the surgical procedure of microfracture. More recently there has been an interest in cell-based strategies for the repair of articular cartilage including autologous chondrocyte implantation (ACI) (Peterson et al 2003), but the results are variable (Lee et al 2000).

A potential alternative source to the use of primary chondrocytes for cell-based cartilage repair strategies, that has been a focus of recent attention, is the use of stem cells or undifferentiated adult progenitor cells. Stem cells possess self-renewal capacity, and exhibit long-term viability and multilineage differentiation potential. In the first instance the alternative stem cell source will potentially be used to replace mature chondrocytes as a cell source in cell-based cartilage repair strategies. The use of stem cells should increase the consistency and reproducibility of the autologous chondrocyte implantation procedure. This could, in the future, be extended to treat more generalised cartilage defects, especially if the cell source is not a limiting factor unlike mature chondrocytes. Cartilage, being an avascular tissue, is an ideal target for tissue engineering.

Tissue engineering applications using MSCs present an interesting and promising new approach for the repair of articular cartilage defects (Hardingham et al, 2002). Mesenchymal stem cells have been shown to differentiate into chondrocytes and represent an alternative cell source for therapeutic repair. Animal studies have successfully reported on the use of bone marrow derived mesenchymal stem cells embedded in a collagen gel to repair chondral defects (Wakitani et al 1994). To date there have been only limited reports of human autologous bone marrow derived cell implantation for cartilage repair (Wakitani et al, 2002; Wakitani, 2005; Kuroda et al, 2007) where expanded cells were embedded within a collagen scaffold, to repair a full-thickness cartilage defect in the knee. In a clinical trial, bone marrow derived mesenchymal stem cells injected into the medial femoral condylar cartilage defects at the time of high tibial osteotomy in twelve patients resulted in clinical improvement compared to the control group where no cells were used (Wakitani et al 2002). Although the score for clinical improvement was not significantly different, the patients treated with bone marrow derived MSCs did have better arthroscopic and histological grading scores. In another study, histological studies suggested that the defect was filled with hyaline-like type of cartilage tissue that stained positively with Safranin-O (Kuroda et al, 2007).

The optimal conditions for chondrogenic differentiation in MSCs derived from various sources are still being developed. We have shown that chondrogenesis in fat pad derived MSCs can be optimised by expanding cells in FGF-2 (Khan et al 2008) and allowing them to differentiate under hypoxic culture conditions (Khan et al 2007).

The management of cartilage defects is currently suboptimal and stem cells have the potential to improve on the current treatment modalities by replacing damaged tissue with hyaline cartilage. Tissue engineering holds promise for the future, but a number of challenges need to be overcome. These include further work on identifying the nature of stem cells and better characterisation, identifying the optimal source of stem cells for cartilage repair, and also identifying conditions that enhance expansion and chondrogenesis. Tissue engineering applications for the repair of cartilage rely on cells, scaffolds and signalling molecules, either in isolation or in combination. The mode of delivery of cells for the repair of articular cartilage will depend on the size of the defect. Smaller well-localised defects can potentially be repaired by the direct injection of cells in the defect similar to current ACI procedures, whereas larger defects would invariably have to rely on an appropriate scaffold similar to current MACI procedures and, with increasing size, also on appropriate signalling molecules. Stem cells could also potentially be used as a vehicle for gene delivery by transfecting cells with recombinant DNA constructs and coding for the expression of certain proteins and growth factors that promote chondrogenesis. In the future the goal is for more biological replacement of the damaged articular cartilage and stem cells have the potential to deliver this goal.

Conclusions

The use of stem cells holds promise for the future, but a number of challenges need to be overcome. Further work is needed to identify the optimal source of stem cells for cartilage repair, and also determine conditions that enhance expansion and chondrogenesis.

Unfortunately most cell surface markers are inadequate in identifying stem cells unambiguously either because these markers are also expressed by non-stem cells, or they are only expressed by stem cells at a particular stage and under particular culture conditions. The exact nature and location of stem cells in any tissue is also not known. It has recently been suggested that bone marrow derived mesenchymal stem cells originate from microvascular pericytes, and, indeed, many of the tissues from which stem cells have been isolated have good vascularisation and they may give a varied source of cells for future treatments.

Once these challenges have been overcome and these questions answered, we can realistically look at using stem cells in patients and expect consistent and good results.

References

[1] Adesida, A. B., Brady, L. M., Khan, W. S. & Hardingham, T. E. (2006). The matrix forming phenotype of human meniscus cells is enhanced by expansion in the presence of fibroblast growth factor 2 and hypoxia. *Arthritis Res Ther.*, *8*, R61.

[2] Ailhaud, G. (1982). Adipose cell differentiation in culture. *Mol Cell Biochem.*, *49*, 17-31.

[3] Akiyama, H., Chaboissier, M. C., Martin, J. F., Schedl, A. & de Crombrugghe, B. (2002). The transcription factor SOX9 has essential roles in successive steps of the chondrocyte differentiation pathway and is required for the expression of SOX5 and SOX6. *Genes Dev.*, *16*, 2813-28.

[4] Alison, M. R., Poulsom, R., Forbes, S. & Wright, N. A. (2002). An introduction to stem cells. *J Path*, *197*, 419-23.

[5] Andreeva, E. R., Pugach, I. M., Gordon, D. & Orekhov, A. N. (1998). Continuous subendothelial network formed by pericyte-like cells in human vascular bed. *Tiss Cell*, *30*, 127-35.

[6] Baddoo, M., Hill, K., Wilkinson, R., Gaupp, D., Hughes, C., Kopen, G. C. & Phinney, D. G. (2003). Characterisation of mesenchymal stem cells isolated from murine bone marrow by negative selection. *J Cell Biochem.*, *89*, 1235-49.

[7] Bankfalvi, A., Terpe, H. J., Breukelmann, D., Bier, B., Rempe, D., Schadka, G., Krech, R. & Bocker, W. (1998). Gains and losses of CD44 expression during breast carcinogenesis and tumour progression. *Histopathology*, *33*, 107-16.

[8] Barry, F. P., Boynton, R. E., Haynesworth, S., Murphy, J. M. & Zaia, J. (1999). The monoclonal antibody SH-2, raised against human mesenchymal stem cells, recognises an epitope on endoglin (CD105). *Biochem Biophys Res Commun*, *265*, 134-9.

[9] Barry, F., Boyton, R., Murphy, M., Haynesworth, S. & Zaia, J. (2001). The SH-3 and SH-4 antibodies recognize distinct epitopes on CD73 from human mesenchymal stem cells. *Biochem Biophys Res Commun*, 289, 519-24.

[10] Bentley, G. & Minas, T. (2000). Treating joint damage in young people. *BMJ.*, *320*, 1585-8.

[11] Bentley, G., Biant, L. C., Carrington, R. W., Akmal, M., Goldberg, A., Williams, A. M., Skinner, J. A. & Pringle, J. (2003). A prospective, randomised comparison of

autologous chondrocyte implantation versus mosaicoplasty for osteochondral defects in the knee. *J Bone Joint Surg Br., 85*, 223-30.

[12] Benya, P. D. & Shaffer, J. D. (1982). Dedifferentiated chondrocytes reexpress the differentiated collagen phenotype when cultured in agarose gels. *Cell, 30*, 215-24.

[13] Beresford, J. N., Joyner, C. J., Devlin, C. & Triffitt, J. T. (1994). The effects of dexamethasone and 1, 25-dihydroxyvitamin D3 on osteogenic differentiation of human marrow stromal cells in vitro. *Arch Oral Biol., 39*, 941-7.

[14] Bertram, H., Mayer, H., Schliephake, H. (2005). Effect of donor characteristics, technique of harvesting and in vitro processing on culturing of human marrow stroma cells for tissue engineered growth of bone. *Clin Oral Implants Res., 16,* 524-31.

[15] Bianchi, G., Banfi, A., Mastrgiacoma, M., Notaro, R., Luzzatto, L., Cancedda, R. & Quarto, R. (2003). Ex vivo enrichment of mesenchymal cell progenitors by fibroblast growth factor 2. *Exp Cell Res., 287*, 98-105.

[16] Bianco, P., Riminucci, M., Gronthos, S. & Robey, P. G. (2001). Bone marrow stromal stem cell: nature, biology and potential applications. *Stem Cells, 19*, 180-92.

[17] Brighton, C.T., Lorich, D.G., Kupcha, R., Reilly, T.M., Jones, A.R., Woodbury, R.A. 2nd (1992). The pericyte as a possible osteoblast progenitor cell. *Clin Orthop Relat Res., 275,* 287-99.

[18] Brittberg, M., Lindahl, A., Nilsson, C., Isaksson, O. & Patterson, L. (1994). Treatment of deep cartilage defects in the knee with autologous chondrocyte transplantation. *N Engl J Med., 331*, 889-95.

[19] Brittberg, M., Tallheden, T., Sjogren-Jansson, B., Lindahl, A. & Peterson, L. (2001). Autologous chondrocytes used for articular cartilage repair: an update. *Clin Orthop, 391*, S337-48.

[20] Brittberg, M., Peterson, L., Sjogren-Jansson, E., Tallheden, T. & Lindahl, A. (2003). Articular cartilage engineering with autologous chondrocyte transplantation. *J Bone Joint Surg Am., 85*, 109-15.

[21] Bruder, S. P., Jaiswal, N. & Haynesworth, S. E. (1997a). Growth kinetics, self renewal and the osteogenic potential of purified human mesenchymal stem cells during extensive subcultivation and following cryopreservation. *J Cell Biochem, 64*, 278-94.

[22] Bruder, S. P., Horowitz, M. C., Mosca, J. D. & Haynesworth, S. E. (1997b). Monoclonal antibodies reactive with human osteogenic cell surface antigens. *Bone, 21*, 225-35.

[23] Bruder, S. P., Ricalton, N. S., Boynton, R. E., Connolly, T. J., Jaiswal, N., Zaia, J. & Barry, F. P. (1998). Mesenchymal stem cell surface antigen SB-10 corresponds to activated leucocyte cell adhesion molecule and is involved in osteogenic differentiation. *J Bone Miner Res., 13*, 655-63.

[24] Buckwalter, J. A. (2002). Articular cartilage injuries. *Clin Orthop Relat Res., 402*, 21-37.

[25] Cancedda, R., Dozin, B., Giannoni, P. & Quarto, R. (2003). Tissue engineering and cell therapy of cartilage and bone. *Matrix Biol., 22*, 81-91.

[26] Chia, S.L., Sawaji, Y., Burleigh, A., McLean, C., Inglis, J., Saklatvala, J., Vincent, T. (2009). Fibroblast growth factor 2 is an intrinsic chondroprotective agent that

suppresses ADAMTS-5 and delays cartilage degradation in murine osteoarthritis. *Arthritis Rheum., 60,* 2019-27.

[27] Clar, C., Cummins, E., McIntyre, L., Thomas, S., Lamb, J., Bain, L., Jobanputra, P. & Waugh, N. (2005). Clinical and cost-effectiveness of autologous chondrocyte implantation for cartilage defects in knee joints: systematic review and economic evaluation. *Health Technol Assess*, *9*, 1-82.

[28] D'Ippolito, G., Schiller, P. C., Ricordi, C., Roos, B. A. & Howard, G. A. (1999). Age related osteogenic potential of mesenchymal stromal stem cells from human vertebral bone marrow. *J Bone Miner Res*., *14*, 1115-22.

[29] De Bari, C., Dell'Accio, F., Tylzanowski, P. & Luyten, F. P. (2001). Multipotent mesenchymal stem cells from adult human synovial membrane. *Arthritis Rheum*, *44*, 1928-42.

[30] Deans, R. J. & Moseley, A. B. (2000). Mesenchymal stem cells: biology and potential clinical uses. *Exp Haematol*, *28*, 875-84.

[31] Dennis, J. E. & Caplan, A. I. (2000). Bone marrow mesenchymal stem cells. *Stem cell handbook by Stewart Sell*, Humana Press.

[32] Dennis, J. E., Carbillet, J. P., Caplan, A. I. & Charbord, P. (2002). The STRO-1+ marrow cell population is multipotential. *Cells Tissues Organs*., *170*, 73-82.

[33] Deren, J. A., Kaplan, F. S. & Brighton, C. T. (1990). Alkaline phosphatase production by periosteal cells at various oxygen tensions in vitro. *Clin Orthop Rel Res*., *252*, 307-12.

[34] de Wert, G. & Mummery, C. (2003). Human embryonic stem cells: research, ethics and policy. *Hum Reprod*, *18*, 672-82.

[35] Devine, S. M. & Hoffman, R. (2000). Role of mesenchymal stem cells in hematopoietic stem cell transplantation. *Curr Opin Hematol*, *7*, 358-63.

[36] Doherty, M., Ashton, B., Walsh, S., Beresford, J., Grant, M. & Canfield, A. (1998). Vascular pericytes express osteogenic potential in vitro and in vivo. *J Bone Miner Res*., *13*, 828-38.

[37] Domm, C., Schunke, M., Christesen, K. & Kurz, B. (2002). Redifferentiation of dedifferentiated bovine articular chondrocytes in alginate culture under low oxygen tension. *Osteoarthritis Cartilage*, *10*, 13-22.

[38] Dozin, B., Malpeli, M., Camardella, L., Cancedda, R. & Pietrangelo, A. (2002). Response of young, aged and osteoarthritic human articular chondrocytes to inflammatory cytokines: molecular and cellular aspects. *Matrix Biol*., *21*, 449-59.

[39] Dragoo, J. L., Samimi, B., Zhu, M., Hame, S. L., Thomas, B. J., Lieberman, J. R., Hedrick, M. H. & Benhaim. P. (2003). Tissue-engineered cartilage and bone using stem cells from human infrapatellar fat pads. *J Bone Joint Surg Br*., *85*, 740-7.

[40] Draper, J. S., Moore, H. D., Ruban, L. N., Gokhale, P. J. & Andrews, P. W. (2004). Culture and characterization of human embryonic stem cells. *Stem Cells Dev*., *13*, 325-36.

[41] Duri, Z. A., Aichroth, P. M. & Dowd, G. (1996). The fat pad: Clinical observations. *Am J Knee Surg*., *9*, 55-66.

[42] Erices, A., Conget, P. & Minguell, J. J. (2000). Mesenchymal progenitor cells in human umbilical cord blood. *Br J Haematol*, *109*, 235-42.

[43] Eyre, D. R. (1991). The collagens of articular cartilage. *Semin Arthritis Rheum*, *21*, 2-11.

[44] Farrington-Rock, C., Crofts, N. J., Doherty, M. J., Ashton, B. A., Griffin-Jones, C. & Canfield, A. E. (2004). Chondrogenic and adipogenic potential of microvascular pericytes. *Circulation*, *110*, 2226-32.

[45] Freidenstein, A. J., Piatetzky, II, S. & Petrakova, K. V. (1966). Osteogenesis in transplants of bone marrow cells. *J Embryol Exp Morphol*, *16*, 381-90.

[46] Freidenstein, A. J., Petrakova, K. V., Kurolesova, A. I. & Frolova, G. P. (1968). Heterotrophic of bone marrow. Analysis of precursoe cells for osteogenic and haematopoietic tissues. *Transplantation*, *6*, 230-47.

[47] Freidenstein, A. J., Chailakhjan, R. K. & Lalykina, K. S. (1970). The development of fibroblast colonies in monolayer cultures of guinea pig bone marrow and spleen cells. *Cell Tissue Kinet*, *4*, 393-403.

[48] Furumatsu, T., Tsuda, M., Taniguchi, N., Tajima, Y. & Asahara, H. (2005). Smad3 induces chondrogenesis through the activation of SOX9 via CREB-binding protein/p300 recruitment. *J Biol Chem.*, *280*, 8343-50.

[49] Garcia-Pacheco, J. M., Oliver, C., Kimatrai, M., Blanco, F. J. & Olivares, E. G. (2001). Human decidual stromal cells express CD34 and STRO-1 and are related to bone marrow stromal precursors. *Mol Hum Reprod*, *7*, 1151-7.

[50] Gregoire, F. M. (2001). Adipocyte differentiation: from fibroblast to endocrine cell. *Exp Biol Med.*, *226*, 997-1002.

[51] Gronthos, S., Graves, S. E., Ohta, S. & Simmons, P. J. (1994). The STRO-1+ fraction of adult human boné marrow contains osteogenic precursors. *Blood*, *84*, 4164-73.

[52] Gronthos, S., Zannettino, A. C., Graves, S. E., Ohta, S., Hay, S. J. & Simmons, P. J. (1999). Differential cell surface expression of the STRO-1 and alkaline phosphatase antigens on discrete developmental stages in primary cultures of human bone cells. *J Bone Miner Res.*, *14*, 47-56.

[53] Gronthos, S., Zanettino, A. C. W., Shelley, J. H., Shi, S., Graves, S. E., Kortesidis, A. & Simmons, P. J. (2003). Molecular and cellular characterization of highly purified stromal stem cells derived from human bone marrow. *J Cell Sci.*, *116*, 1827-35.

[54] Hardingham, T.E., Fosang, A.J. (1992). Proteoglycans: many forms and many functions. *FASEB J.*, *6*, 861-70.

[55] Hardingham, T. E. (1998). Pathophysiology of musculoskeletal disease. In Oxford Textbook of Rheumatology. Maddison, P. J., Isenberg, D. A., Woo, P. & Glass, D. N. Eds. *Second edition Oxford Medical Publications*, 1-10.

[56] Hardingham, T., Tew, S. & Murdoch, A. (2002). Tissue engineering: chondrocytes and cartilage. *Arthritis Res.*, *4*, S63-8.

[57] Haynesworth, S. E., Baber, M. A. & Caplan, A. I. (1992). Cell surface antigen on human marrow derived mesenchymal cells are detected by monoclonal antibodies. *Bone*, *13*, 69-80.

[58] Herman, I. M. & D'Amore, P. A. (1985). Microvascular pericytes contain muscle and nonmuscle actins. *J Cell Biol.*, *101*, 43-52.

[59] Hiraki, Y., Shukunami, C., Iyama, K. & Mizuta, H. (2001). Differentiation of chondrogenic precursor cells during the regeneration of articular cartilage. *Osteoarthritis Cartilage*, *9*, S102-8.

[60] Hirschi, K. K. & D'Amore, P. A. (1996). Pericytes in the microvasculature. *Cardiovasc Res.*, *32*, 687-98.

[61] Hirschi, K. K. & D'Amore, P. A. (1997). Control of angiogenesis by the pericyte: molecular mechanisms and significance. *EXS.*, *79*, 419-28.

[62] Homicz, M. R., Schumacher, B. L., Sah, R. L. & Watson, D. (2002). Effects of serial expansion of septal chondrocytes on tissue-engineered neocartilage composition. *Otolaryngol Head Neck Surg.*, *127*, 398-408.

[63] Huang, J. I., Kazmi, N., Durbhakula, M. M., Hering, T. M., Yoo, J. U. & Johnstone, B. (2005). Chondrogenic potential of progenitor cells derived from human bone marrow and adipose tissue: A patient matched comparison. *J Orthop Res.*, *23*, 1383-9.

[64] Hunziker, E. B. (2001). Articular cartilage repair: basic science and clinical progress; a review of the current status and prospects. *Osteoarthritis Cartilage*, *10*, 432-63.

[65] Indrawattana, N., Chen, G., Tadokoro, M., Shann, L. H., Ohgushi, H., Tateishi, T., Tanaka, J. & Bunyaratvej, A. (2004). Growth factor combination for chondrogenic induction from human mesenchymal stem cell. *Biochem Biophys Res Commun.*, *320*, 914-9.

[66] Ishino, T., Hirakawa, K., Takeno, S., Furukido, K., Sugimoto, I. & Yajin, K. (2004). Bone-constructing cells from ethmoid bone may have multilineage differentiation potential: preliminary report. *Acta Otolaryngol Suppl.*, *553*, 105-8.

[67] Jiang, Y., Mishima, H., Sakai, S., Liu, Y, K., Ohyabu, Y., Uemura, T. (2008). Gene expression analysis of major lineage-defining factors in human bone marrow cells: effect of aging, gender, and age-related disorders. *J Orthop Res.*, *26*, 910-7.

[68] Johnstone, B., Hering, T. M., Caplan, A. I., Goldberg, V. M. & Yoo, J. U. (1998). In vitro chondrogenesis of bone marrow-derived mesenchymal progenitor cells. *Exp Cell Res.*, *238*, 265-72.

[69] Jones, E. A., Kinsey, S. E., English, A., Jones, R. A., Straszynski, L., Meredith, D. M., Markham, A. F., Jack, A., Emery, P. & McGonagle, D. (2002). Isolation and characterisation of bone marrow multipotential mesenchymal progenitor cells. *Arthritis Rheum*, *46*, 3349-60.

[70] Jones, E. A., English, A., Henshaw, K., Kinsey, S. E., Markham, A. F., Emery, P. & McGonagle, D. (2004). Enumeration and phenotypic characterisation of synovial fluid multipotential mesenchymal progenitor cells in inflammatory and degenerative arthritis. *Arthritis Rheum*, *50*, 817-27.

[71] Karsenty, G. & Wagner, E. F. (2002). Reaching a genetic and molecular understanding of skeletal development. *Dev Cell*, *2*, 389-406.

[72] Kato, Y. & Gospodarowicz, D. (1985). Sulfated proteoglycan synthesis by confluent cultures of rabbit costal chondrocytes grown in the presence of fibroblast growth factor. *J Cell Biol.*, *100*, 477-85.

[73] Khan, W. S., Adesida, A. B., Hardingham, T. E. (2007). Hypoxic conditions increase hypoxia-inducible transcription factor 2alpha and enhance chondrogenesis in stem cells from the infrapatellar fat pad of osteoarthritis patients. *Arthritis Res Ther.*, *9*, R55.

[74] Khan, W. S., Tew, S. R., Adesida, A. B., Hardingham, T. E. (2008). Human infrapatellar fat pad-derived stem cells express the pericyte marker 3G5 and show enhanced chondrogenesis after expansion in fibroblast growth factor-2. *Arthritis Res Ther., 10,* R74.

[75] Khan, W. S., Adesida, A. B., Tew, S. R., Hardingham, T. E. The epitope characterisation and osteogenic differentiation potential of fat pad derived stem cells is maintained with ageing in later life. *Injury* (in press).

[76] Kim, S. J., Min, B. H. & Kim, H. K. (1996). Arthroscopic anatomy of the infrapatellar plica. *Arthroscopy*, *12*, 561-4.

[77] Kohn, D., Deiler, S. & Rudert, M. (1995). Arterial blood supply of the infrapatellar fat pad. Anatomy and clinical consequences. *Arch Orthop Trauma Surg.*, *114*, 72-5.

[78] Koller, M. R., Bender, J. G., Papoutsakis, E. T. & Miller, W. M. (1992). Effects of synergistic cytokine combinations, low oxygen, and irradiated stroma on the expansion of human cord blood progenitors. *Blood*, *80*, 403-11.

[79] Krampera, M., Glennie, S., Dyson, J., Scott, D., Laylor, R., Simpson, E. & Dazzi, F. (2003). Bone marrow mesenchymal stem cells inhibit the response of naive and memory antigen-specific T cells to their cognate peptide. *Blood*, *101*, 3722-9.

[80] Kuroda, R., Isada, K., Matsumoto, T., Akisue, T., Fujioka, H., Mizuno, K., Ohgushi, H., Wakitani, S., Kurosaka, M. (2007). Treatment of a full-thickness articular cartilage defect in the femoral condyle of an athlete with autologous bone-marrow stromal cells. *Osteoarthritis Cartilage., 15,* 226-31.

[81] La Prade, R. F. (1998). The anatomy of the deep infrapatellar bursa of the knee. *Am J Sports Med.*, *26*, 129-32.

[82] Le Blanc, K., Rasmusson, I., Sundberg, B., Götherström, C., Hassan, M., Uzunel, M., Ringdén, O. (2004). Treatment of severe acute graft-versus-host disease with third party haploidentical mesenchymal stem cells. *Lancet., 363,* 1439-41.

[83] Lee, C. R., Grodzinsky, A. J., Hsu, H. P., Martin, S. D. & Spector, M. (2000). Effects of harvest and selected cartilage repair procedures on the physical and biochemical properties of articular cartilage in the canine knee. *J Orthop Res.*, *18*, 790-9.

[84] Lennon, D. P., Edmison, J. M. & Caplan, A. I. (2001). Cultivation of rat marrow-derived mesenchymal stem cells in reduced oxygen tension: effects on in vitro and in vivo osteochondrogenesis. *J Cell Physiol*, *187*, 345-55.

[85] Li, Y., Tew, S. R., Russel, A. M., Gonzalez, K. R., Hardingham, T. E. & Hawkins, R. E. (2004). Transduction of passaged human articular chondrocytes with adenoviral, retroviral, and lentiviral vectors and the effects of enhanced expression of SOX9. *Tissue Eng.*, *10*, 575-84.

[86] Loty, S., Forest, N., boulekbache, H. & Sautier, J. M. (1995). Cytochalasin D induces changes in cell shape and promotes in vitro chondrogenesis: a morphological study. *Biol Cell*, *83*, 149-61.

[87] MacDougald, O. A. & Mandrup, S. (2002). Adipogenesis: forces that tip the scales. *Trends Endocrinol Metab*,*13*, 5-11.

[88] Mackay, A. M., Beck, S. C., Murphy, J. M., Barry, F. P., Chichester, C. O. & Pittenger, M. F. (1998). Chondrogenic differentiation of cultured marrow mesenchymal stem cells from marrow. *Tissue Eng.*, *4*, 415-28.

[89] Magne, D., Vinatier, C., Julien, M., Weiss, P. & Guicheux, J. (2005a). Mesenchymal stem cell therapy to rebuild cartilage. *Trends Mol Med., 11*, 519-26

[90] Magne, D., Julien, M., Vinatier, C., Merhi-Soussi, F., Weiss, P. & Guicheux, J. (2005b). Cartilage formation in growth plate and arteries: from physiology to pathology. *Bioessays, 27*, 708-16.

[91] Majumdar, M. K., Keane-Moore, M., Buyaner, D., Hardy, W. B., Moorman, M. A., McIntosh, K. R. & Mosca, J. D. (2003). Characterization and functionality of cell surface molecules on human mesenchymal stem cells. *J Biomed Sci., 10*, 228-41.

[92] Manne, U., Srivastava, R. G. & Srivastava, S. (2005). Recent advances in biomarkers for cancer diagnosis and treatment. *Drug Discov Today, 10*, 965-76.

[93] Mareschi, K., Ferrero, I., Rustichelli, D., Aschero, S., Gammaitoni, L., Aglietta, M., Madon, E., Fagioli, F. (2006). Expansion of mesenchymal stem cells isolated from paediatric and adult donor bone marrow. *J Cell Biochem., 97,* 744-54.

[94] Martin, I., Muraglia, A., Campanile, G., Cancedda, R. & Quarto, R. (1997). Fibroblast growth factor-2 supports ex vivo expansion and maintenance of osteogenic precursors from human bone marrow. *Endocrinology, 138*, 4456-62.

[95] Martin, J. A. & Buckwalter, J. A. (2003). The role of chondrocyte senescence in the pathogenesis of osteoarthritis and in limiting cartilage repair. *J Bone Joint Surg Am., 85*, S106-10.

[96] Meyrick, B., Fujiwara, K. & Reid, L. (1981). Smooth muscle myosin in precursor and mature smooth muscle cells in normal pulmonary arteries and the effect of hypoxia. *Exp Lung Res., 2*, 303-13.

[97] Miranville, A., Heeschen, C., Sengenes, C., Curat, C. A., Busse, R. & Bouloumie, A. (2004). Improvement of postnatal neovascularisation by human adipose tissue derived stem cells. *Circulation, 110*, 349-55.

[98] Mochizuki, T., Muneta, T., Sakaguchi, Y., Nimura, A., Yokoyama, A., Koga, H. & Sekiya, I. (2006). Higher chondrogenic potential of fibrous synovium- and adipose synovium- derived cells compared with subcutaneous fat- derived cells. *Arthritis Rheum, 54*, 843-53.

[99] Morrison, S. J., Csete, M., Groves, A. K., Melega, W., Wold, B. & Anderson, D. J. (2000). Culture in reduced levels of oxygen promotes clonogenic sympathoadrenal differentiation by isolated neural crest stem cells. *J Neurosci, 20*, 7370-6.

[100] Murphy, C. L. & Sambanis, A. (2001). Effect of oxygen tension and alginate encapsulation on restoration of the differentiated phenotype of passaged chondrocytes. *Tissue Eng., 7*, 791-803.

[101] Nayak, R. C., Berman, A. B., George, K. L., Eisenbarth, G. S. & King, G. L. (1988). A monoclonal antibody (3G5) defined ganglioside antigen is expressed on the cell surface of microvascular pericytes. *J Exp Med., 167*, 1003-15.

[102] Newman, A. (1998). Articular cartilage repair. *Am J Sports Med., 26*, 309-24.

[103] Nishida, S., Endo, N., Yamagiwa, H., Tanizawa, T. & Takahashi, H. E. (1999). Number of osteoprogenitor cells in human bone marrow markedly decreases after skeletal maturation. *J Bone Miner Metab, 17*, 171-7.

[104] O'Driscoll, S. W. (1998). The healing and regeneration of articular cartilage. *J Bone Joint Surg Am., 80*, 1795-812.

[105] Ogilvie-Harris, D. J. & Giddens, J. (1994). Hoffa's disease: arthroscxopic resection of the infrapatellar fat pad. *Arthroscopy, 10*, 184-7.

[106] Orkin, SH. & Morrison, S. J. (2002). Stem-cell competition. *Nature, 418*, 25-7.

[107] Owen, M. E., Cave, J. & Joyner, C. J. (1987). Clonal analysis in vitro of osteogenic differentiation of marrow CFU-F. *J Cell Sci., 87*, 731-8.

[108] Owen, M. & Friedenstein, A. J. (1988). Stromal stem cells: marrow-derived osteogenic precursors. *Ciba Found Symp., 136*, 42-60.

[109] Parsons, I. M. & Sonnabend, D. H. (2004). What is the role of joint replacement surgery? *Best Pract Res Clin Rheumatol, 18*, 557-72.

[110] Peng, H. & Huard, J. (2003). Stem cells in the treatment of muscle and connective tissue diseases. *Curr Opin Pharmacol, 3*, 329-33.

[111] Peterson, L., Minas, T., Brittberg, M., Lindahl, A. (2003). Treatment of osteochondritis dissecans of the knee with autologous chondrocyte transplantation: results at two to ten years. *J Bone Joint Surg., 85A,* 17-24.

[112] Pittenger, M. F., Mackay, A. M., Beck, S. C., Jaiswal, R. K., Douglas, R., Mosca, J. D., Moorman, M. A., Simonetti, D. W., Craig, S. & Marshak, D. R. (1999). Multilineage potential of adult human mesenchymal stem cells. *Science, 284*, 143-7.

[113] Pittenger, M. F., Mbalaviele, G., Black, M., Mosca, J. D. & Marshak, D. R. (2001). Mesenchymal stem cells. In: Koller MR., Palsson BO., Masters JRW Eds. Primary mesenchymal cells. Dordrecht; Boston: *Kluwer Academic Publishers*, : 189-207.

[114] Pittinger, M. F. & Martin, B. J. (2004). Mesenchymal stem cells and their potential as cardiac therapeutics. *Circ Res., 95*, 9-20.

[115] Poole, A. R. (1995). Imbalance of anabolism and catabolism of cartilage matrix componenets in osteoarthritis. In: Kuettner, K. E. & Goldberg, B. Eds. Osteoarthritic disorders. Rosemont: *AAOS*, 247-60.

[116] Prockop, D. J. (1997). Marrow stromal cells as stem cells for nonhaematopoietic tissues. *Science, 276*, 71-4.

[117] Qiu, Z., Wei, Y., Chen, N., Jiang, M., Wu, J. & Liao, K. (2001). DNA synthesis and mitotic clonal expansion is not a required step for 3T3–L1 preadipocyte differentiation into adipocytes. *J Biol Chem., 276*, 11988-95.

[118] Quirici, N., Soligo, D., Bossolasco, P., Servida, F., Lumini, C. & Deliliers, G. L. (2002). Isolation of bone marrow mesenchymal stem cells by anti-nerve growth factor receptor antibodies. *Exp Haematol, 30*, 783-91.

[119] Raghunath, J., Salacinski, H. J., Sales, K. M., Butler, P. E. & Seifalian, M. (2005). Advancing cartilage tissue engineering: the application of stem cell technology. *Curr Opin Biotech, 16*, 503-9.

[120] Ramirez-Zacarias, J. L., Castro-Munozledo, F. & Kuri-Harcuch, W. (1992). Quantitation of adipose conversion and triglycerides by staining intracytoplasmic lipids with Oil red O. *Histochem, 97*, 493-7.

[121] Rhodin, J. A. (1968). Ultrastructure of mammalian venous capillaries, venules, and small collecting veins. *J Ultrastruct Res., 25*, 452-500.

[122] Rich, I. N. & Kubanek, B. (1982). The effect of reduced oxygen tension on colony formation of erythropoietic cells in vitro. *Br J Haematol, 52*, 579-88.

[123] Rich, I. N. (1986). A role for the macrophage in normal hemopoiesis. II. Effect of varying physiological oxygen tensions on the release of hemopoietic growth factors from bone marrow derived macrophages in vitro. *Exp Haematol, 14*, 746-51.

[124] Rim, J. S., Mynatt, R. L. & Gawronska-Kozak, B. (2005). Mesenchymal stem cells from the outer ear: a novel adult stem cell model system for the study of adipogenesis. *FASEB J. 19*, 1205-7.

[125] Risbud, M. V. & Sittinger, M. (2002). Tissue engineering: advances in in vitro cartilage generation. *Trends Biotech, 20*, 351-6.

[126] Rosen, E. D. & Spiegelman, B. M. (2000). Molecular regulation of adipogenesis. *Annu Rev Cell Dev Biol., 16*, 145-71.

[127] Saddik, D., McNally, E. G. & Richardson, M. (2004). MRI of Hoffa's fat pad. *Skeletal Radiol, 33*, 433-44

[128] Sakaguchi, Y., Sekiya, I., Yagishita, K. & Muneta, T. (2005). Comparison of human stem cells derived from various mesenchymal tissues- Superiority of synovium as a cell source. *Arthritis Rheum, 52*, 2521-9.

[129] Scharstuhl, A., Schewe, B., Benz, K., Gaissmaier, C., Bühring, H. J., Stoop, R. (2007). Chondrogenic potential of human adult mesenchymal stem cells is independent of age or osteoarthritis etiology. *Stem Cells., 25,* 3244-51.

[130] Scherer, K., Schunke, M., Sellckau, R., Hassenpflug, J. & Kurz, B. (2004). The influence of oxygen and hydrostatic pressure on articular chondrocytes and adherent bone marrow cells in vitro. *Biorheology, 41*, 323-33.

[131] Schipani, E., Ryan, H. E., Didrickson, S., Kobayashi, T., Knight, M. & Johnson, R. S. (2001). Hypoxia in cartilage: HIF1 is essential for chondrocyte growth arrest and survival. *Genes Dev., 15*, 2865-76

[132] Schipper, B. M., Marra, K. G., Zhang, W., Donnenberg, A. D., Rubin, J. P. (2008). Regional anatomic and age effects on cell function of human adipose-derived stem cells. *Ann Plast Surg., 60,* 538-44.

[133] Schulz, R. M., Bader, A. (2007). Cartilage tissue engineering and bioreactor systems for the cultivation and stimulation of chondrocytes. *Eur Biophys J., 36,* 539-68.

[134] Sekiya, I., Vuoristo, J. T., Larson, B. L. & Prockop, D. J. (2002). In vitro cartilage formation by human adult stem cells from bone marrow stroma defines the sequence of cellular and molecular events during chondrogenesis. *Proc Natl Acad Sci U S A, 99,* 4397-402.

[135] Shamsul, B. S., Aminuddin, B. S., Ng, M. H., Ruszymah, B. H. (2004). Age and gender effect on the growth of bone marrow stromal cells in vitro. *Med J Malaysia., 59,* 196-7.

[136] Shapiro, F., Koide, S. & Glimcher, M. J. (1993). Cell origin and differentiation in the repair of full thickness defects of articular cartilage. *J Bone Joint Surg Am., 75*, 532-53.

[137] Shi, S. & Gronthos, S. (2003). Perivascular niche of postnatal mesenchymal stem cells in human bone marrow and dental pulp. *J Bone Miner Res., 18*, 696-704.

[138] Short, B., Brouard, N., Occhioduro-Scott, T., Ramakrishnand, A. & Simmons, P. J. (2003). Mesenchymal stem cells. *Arch Med Res., 34*, 565-71.

[139] Siddappa, R., Licht, R., van Blitterswijk, C., de Boer, J. (2007). Donor variation and loss of multipotency during in vitro expansion of human mesenchymal stem cells for bone tissue engineering. *J Orthop Res., 25,* 1029-41.

[140] Silver, I. A. (1975). Measurement of pH and ionic composition of pericellular sites. *Philos Trans R Soc Lond B Biol Sci.*, *271*, 261-72.

[141] Simmons, P. J. & Torok-Storb, B. (1991). Identification of stromal cell prcursors in human bone marrow by a novel monoclonal antibody, STRO-1. *Blood*, *78*, 55-62.

[142] Simon, L. (1999). Osteoarthritis: a review. *Clin Cornerstone*, *2*, 26-37.

[143] Smillie, I. S. (1974). *Disease of the knee joint*, 1st edn. London: Churchill Livingstone.

[144] Solchaga, L. A., Penick, K., Porter, J. D., Goldberg, V. M., Caplan, A. I. & Welter, J. F. (2005). FGF-2 enhances the mitotic and chondrogenic potentials of human adult bone marrow-derived mesenchymal stem cells. *J Cell Physiol*, *203*, 398-409.

[145] Sottile, V. & Seuwen, K. (2001). A high capacity screen for adipogenic differentiation. *Anal Biochem*, *293*, 124-8.

[146] Spees, J. L., Gregory, C. A., Singh, H., Tucker, H. A., Peister, A., Lynch, P. J., Hsu, S. C., Smith, J. & Prockop, D. J. (2004). Internalised antigens must be removed to prepare hypoimmunogenic mesenchymal stem cells for cell and gene therapy. *Mol Ther.*, *9*, 747-56.

[147] Stenderup, K., Justesen, J., Clausen, C. & Kassem, M. (2003). Aging is associated with decreased maximal life span and accelerated senescence of bone marrow stromal cells. *Bone*, *33*, 919-26.

[148] Stewart, K., Walsh, S., Screen, J., Jefferiss, C. M., Chainey, J., Jordan, G. R. & Beresford, J. N. (1999). Further characterisation of cells expressing STRO-1 in cultures of adult human bone marrow stromal cells. *J Bone Miner Res.*, *14*, 1345-56.

[149] Stolzing, A., Jones, E., McGonagle, D., Scutt, A. (2008). Age-related changes in human bone marrow-derived mesenchymal stem cells: consequences for cell therapies. *Mech Ageing Dev., 129,* 163-73.

[150] Suva, D., Garavaglia, G., Menetrey, J., Chapuis, B., Hoffmeyer, P., Bernheim, L., Kindler, V. (2004). Non-hematopoietic human bone marrow contains long-lasting, pluripotential mesenchymal stem cells. *J Cell Physiol., 198,* 110-8.

[151] Tew, S. R., Hardingham, T. E. (2006). Regulation of SOX9 mRNA in Human Articular Chondrocytes Involving p38 MAPK Activation and mRNA Stabilization. *J Biol Chem., 281,* 39471-9.

[152] Thomas, W. E. (1999). Brain macrophages: on the role of pericytes and perivascular cells. *Brain Res Brain Res Rev.*, *31*, 42-57.

[153] Thomson, J. A., Itskovitz-Eldor, J., Shapiro, S. S., Waknitz, M. A., Swiergiel, J. J., Marshall, V. S. & Jones, J. M. (1998). Embryonic stem cell lines derived from human blastocysts. *Science*, *282*, 1145-7.

[154] Triffitt, J. T. (2002). Stem cells and the philosopher's stone. *J Cell Biochem Suppl*, *38*, 38, 13-9.

[155] Vaananen, H. K. (2005). Mesenchymal stem cells. *Ann Med.*, *37*, 469-79.

[156] Vats, A., Tolley, N. S., Bishop, A. E. & Polak, J. M. (2005). Embryonic stem cells and tissue engineering: delivering stem cells to the clinic. *J R Soc Med.*, *98*, 346-50.

[157] Wakitani, S., Goto, T., Pineda, S. J., Young, R. G., Mansour, J. M., Caplan, A. I. & Goldberg, V. M. (1994). Mesenchymal cell-based repair of large, full-thickness defects of articular cartilage. *J Bone Joint Surg Am.*, *76*, 579-92.

[158] Wang, D. W., Fermor, B., Gimble, J. M., Awad, H. A. & Guilak, F. (2005). Influence of oxygen on the proliferation and metabolism of adipose derived adult stem cells. *J Cell Physiol.*, *204*, 184-91.

[159] Watt, F. M. (1988). Effect of seeding density on stability of the differentiated phenotype of pig articular chondrocytes in culture. *J Cell Sci.*, *89*, 373-8.

[160] Wesseling, P., Schlingemann, R. O., Rietveld, F. J., Link, M., Burger, P. C. & Ruth, D. J. (1995). Early and extensive contribution of pericytes/ vascular smooth muscle cells to microvascular proliferation in glioblastoma multiforme: an immuno-light and immuno-electron microscopy study. *J Neuropathol Exp Neurol*, *54*, 304-10

[161] Wickham, M. Q., Erickson, G. R., Gimble, J. M., Vail, T. P. & Guilak, F. (2003). Multipotent stromal cells derived from the infrapatellar fat pad of the knee. *Clin Orthop*, *412*, 196-212.

[162] Williams, P., Warwick, R. & Dyson, M. et al (1989). Gray's Anatomy, 37th edn. New York: Churchill Livingstone.

[163] Wollheim, F. (1996). Current pharmacological treatments of osteoarthritis. *Drugs*, *52*, 27-38.

[164] Wroblewski, J. & Edwall-Arvidsson, C. (1995). Inhibitory effects of basic fibroblast growth factor on chondrocyte differentiation. *J Bone Miner Res.*, *10*, 735-42.

[165] Zhou, G., Garofalo, S., Mukhopadhyay, K., Lefebvre, V., Smith, C. N., Eberspaecher, H. & de Crombrugghe, B. (1995). A 182 bp fragment of the mouse pre alpha 1 (II) collagen gene is sufficient to direct chondrocyte expression in transgenic mice. *J Cell Sci.*, *108*, 3677-84.

[166] Zuk, P. A., Zhu, M., Mizino, H., Huang, J., Futrell, J. W., Katz, A. J., Benhaim, P., Lorenz, H. P. & Hedrick, M. H. (2001). Multilineage cells from human adipose tissue: implications for cell-based therapies. *Tissue Eng.*, *7*, 211-28.

[167] Zuk, P. A., Zhu, M., Ashjian, P., De Ugarte, D. A., Huang, J. I., Mizino, H., Alfonso, Z. C., Fraser, J. K., Benhaim, P. & Hedrick, M. H. (2002). Human adipose tissue is a source of multipotent stem cells. *Mol Biol Cell.*, *13*, 4279-95.

In: Hand Surgery: Preoperative Expectations...
Editor: Robert H. Beckingsworth
ISBN: 978-1-60876-280-4

Chapter 2

Patient-Completed Regional Outcome Measures in Hand Surgery

***Wasim S Khan*[1*]*, Kalum De Silva*[1]
and Matthew A Ravenscroft[2]**
[1]University College London Institute of Orthopaedics and Musculoskeletal Sciences, Royal National Orthopaedic Hospital, Stanmore, London, HA7 4LP, UK
[2]Department of Trauma and Orthopaedics, Stockport NHS Foundation Trust, Stepping Hill Hospital, Stockport, SK2 7JE, UK

Abstract

Injuries and disease commonly affect the hand and these can significantly affect the ability of an individual to perform activities of daily living. The use of regional outcome measures or scoring systems is important as it allows comparison between these injuries and disease, and allows clinicians to assess progression and the effects of different treatment modalities. A patient-completed questionnaire is efficient in terms of time and resources, and allows the assessment of outcome without the need to attend an outpatient clinic.

It is important that the scoring system allows satisfactory regional outcome measurements specific for the hand. This is particularly important in injuries and disease that involve both upper and lower limbs. The validity, reliability, responsiveness and bias are used for the assessment of various questionnaires. The validity establishes whether the outcome measure actually measures what it was designed to. The criterion, construct, and content or face validity provide various assessment parameters that allow a complete picture of the validity of a questionnaire to be established. An outcome tool has test-retest reproducibility if the same result is obtained when tested at different time points once the

* Corresponding Author: Mr Wasim S Khan, Academic Clinical Fellow, University College London Institute of Orthopaedics and Musculoskeletal Science, Royal National Orthopaedic Hospital, Stanmore, London, HA7 4LP, UK Telephone number: +44 (0) 7791 025554 Fax number: +44 (0) 20 8570 3864 E-mail address: wasimkhan@doctors.org.uk

condition has stabilised. The responsiveness is the ability to detect clinically important changes in disability at various intervals. The effect size and the standardised response mean are used to evaluate the responsiveness. Bias can occur when assumed independent variables such as age, gender, hand dominance or dominant side injured affect responses. There are also many practical issues concerning the use of questionnaires including feasibility of use for the patient and the clinician.

The Disability of the Arm, Shoulder and Hand (DASH) questionnaire, the Patient Evaluation Measure (PEM) questionnaire, and the Michigan Hand Outcome (MHO) questionnaire are a few of the region-specific outcome measures commonly used for the hand, and are patient-completed questionnaires. They are frequently used to assess self-reported patient outcome in orthopaedics, rheumatology and neurology. In this chapter, the validity, reliability, responsiveness and bias of the various questionnaires used for the assessment of the hand will be discussed.

Quesionnaires as Regional Outcome Measures

Why Use Regional Outcome Measures

Injuries and disease commonly affect the hand as it is in regular use. Hand injuries alone account for almost a fifth of all accident and emergency department attendances. The last decade has seen a significant increase in different therapies, operative and non-operative in the management of diseases and injuries of the hand. These injuries and disease are expensive and associated with increasing costs. This is because they can significantly affect the ability of an individual to perform activities of daily living, and have significant socio-economic consequences. Direct costs of these injuries and disease are associated costs associated with the actual therapy. Indirect costs are those associated with the burden on the patient from time off work and lost income, and burden on the wider society from the loss of productivity.

The use of regional outcome measures or scoring systems is important as it not only allows comparison between these injuries and disease, but also allows clinicians to assess progression and the effects of different therapies (Currens, 2000). They are used in routine patient care, clinical audit and research, population surveys and epidemiological studies, resource allocation and assessing the quality of healthcare.

Regional outcome measures exist in many forms and allow the measure of outcome following injury, disease and therapy, and at various intervals. Over the last decade, there has been a shift in outcome measurements from objective measurements made by the clinician to subjective reporting by the patient. It allows a comparison to be made that would justify a change in therapy. With a greater trend of measuring outcome to justify intervention, and its cost implications, it is likely that the use of regional outcome measures will continue to increase.

To identify the effect of these disease and injuries and the effect of various therapies, reliable and valid instruments are required to evaluate any differences. These instruments could also be used to predict the outcomes of different therapies. There is currently no standardised or universally accepted evaluation instrument for the hand (Bucher & Hume, 2002). Although goniometers and dynamometers are routinely used in clinical practice, they only assess structure and function. There is no standard instrument to assess limitation of activities in patients with limited hand function.

Questionnaires as Regional Outcome Measures

The use of questionnaires for data collection in hand surgery, and in all other healthcare disciplines has increased in recent years. Questionnaires allow the collection of data in a standardised manner. With increasing emphasis on evidence-based practice, it is becoming increasingly important to collect data on injuries and disease, and evaluate the effectiveness of various therapies. Questionnaires consist of a series of questions or statements that the patients respond to. These responses are then converted to numeral form and statistically analysed. Questionnaires have many advantages over other regional outcome measures. They take little time to complete, have fewer associated costs and are generally easy to analyse (Bowling, 1997).

Patient-completed disease-specific questionnaires for the hand include the Australian/Canadian Osteoarthritis (AUSCAN) Hand Index. Regional outcome measures are relevant to potentially all pathologies within that region, unlike disease-specific questionnaires that are only relevant to a particular pathology. Although disease-specific questionnaires are more responsive due to the focussed questions, they are limited in their applicability to only a single disorder.

There Patient Outcome of Surgery- Hand/ Arm (POS-Hand/ Arm) is not a disease-specific questionnaire, but for evaluating outcomes in surgery for hand and arm disorders (Cano et al, 2004). It has a greater scope than disease-specific questionnaires but it nevertheless is limited compared to other regional outcome measures as it can not be used in certain circumstances. A large number of hand diseases and injuries are managed non-operatively making the POS-Hand/ Arm irrelevant. It would also not be applicable when trying to ascertain the impact of physiotherapy. Furthermore the developers of the questionnaire designed it with the aim of specifically targeting elective non-malignant surgery.

Why Use Patient-Completed Questionnaires

Patient-completed questionnaires are being increasingly favoured in medical research although there is little evidence to suggest that they are more valid than clinician-completed questionnaires. Patient-completed questionnaires have many advantages over clinician-completed questionnaires. One of the most important factors is cost. Patient-completed questionnaires save time as they can be completed by the patient in the waiting room or at home. The clinician-completed questionnaire on the other hand takes time away from the clinician, and slows down the consultation and the clinic. Telephone questionnaires do reduce the costs associated with clinician-completed questionnaires but they do not negate many of the other disadvantages. In a study comparing the results of health surveys, it was noted that patients were more likely to report health problems in patient-completed questionnaires than in clinician-completed questionnaires (Cook et al, 1993).

Clinician-completed questionnaires can be useful as they can result in a higher response rate and fewer omissions from the questionnaire. They may result in a more thorough consultation, and more information and clarification on particular questions can be made available to the patient. This however may not always be the case as the questionnaire may not be completed by the clinician or the clinician looking after the patient, particularly in blinded studies. Patient-completed questionnaires, by virtue of their design, aim to be clear and concise avoiding the need for further explanation by the clinician.

Patient-completed questionnaires also have the advantage of letting the patient complete the questionnaire at their leisure, and they do not feel rushed into providing just any answer. They do not result in answer bias that could be a feature in clinician-completed questionnaires if the clinician conducting the questionnaire has not received the relevant training to use the questionnaire. Postal questionnaires are cheaper than interview or telephone completed questionnaires, and evidence suggests that patients are more likely to report poorer health states.

Why Use Fixed-Response Questions

The responses for the questions in the patient-completed questionnaires could be in many formats. Fixed-response questions are generally preferred as they allow categorisation of the response. There are many types of scales that are available including the frequency scales, thurstone scales, guttman scales and Likert scales. Frequency scales are numerical and establish how often an event occurs. Thurston scales use empirical data to ensure clinical features being measured are spaced along a continuum. Gutman scales are hierarchical where a higher category response suggests agreement with all lower category responses. Likert scales assume a linear response and a choice of four to nine responses are available between on a continuum from strongly agree to strongly disagree.

At one extreme, only two possible responses exist. At the other extreme, the patients may be presented with a line and chose a response between two extremes i.e. the visual analogue scale. The two possible responses can be frustrating for the patient who fail to better express themselves, and are not much use to the clinician as they do not provide any additional information to enable a more thorough assessment. These two extremes have been falling out of favour and now there is a greater tendency to provide patients with between four and nine fixed responses to chose from. In a study, a seven fixed-response questionnaire was found to be as responsive as the visual analogue score, and easier to administer and interpret. The data generates scores that are used as interval data and allow the use of parametric tests.

It is important however that the fixed responses are logical, avoid overlap and cover the likely response range. There is potential to skew data if the likely response range is not covered appropriately within the categories. There is controversy regarding the provision of a neutral point, as if it was removed it would force the patient to choose a response.

Close-Ended and Open-Ended Questions

Questionnaires usually comprise of closed questions. Open-ended questions may allow the patient to express themselves better, but are difficult for clinicians to analyse. The responses tend to be highly subjective and may not address the issues that the questionnaire wants to address. It is unusual however to see questionnaires with only open-ended questions, and many questionnaires have fixed-response questions with the option of an open-ended question at the end. In such cases it can be useful for the patient by allowing them to better express themselves. They also allow the expression of concerns that would have been brought up in a consultation during a clinician-completed questionnaire. It also allows the clinician to gain insight into the patients' responses. The open-ended questions have an important role in the developing of a questionnaire, but not particularly so in a well-developed questionnaire.

Why Use Domains with More than One Question

Domains are areas of interest that are covered by the questionnaire. In hand questionnaires they tend to be pain, function etc. In many questionnaires there are predetermined domains e.g. pain, function etc, and one or more questions for each domain. It is usual to have more than one question for each domain as it allows a more thorough assessment of each domain. They reduce bias, misinterpretation and reduce measurement error, and they have been shown to be more reliable (Streiner & Norman, 1994). Symptoms like pain and function are complex and multifaceted, and one question alone is generally insufficient to satisfactorily assess them. A number of questions would allow a more thorough assessment of the domain and reduce the chances of bias due to a single answer. It is however important that all questions within the domain are relevant to that domain and are internally consistent.

In the creation of questionnaires first domains are identified and likely questions for each domain are gathered. This is done in a variety of ways. It is commonly done by conducting interviews with patient groups, with an expert panel of clinicians or both. It could also be done by a literature review. This results in a number of questions, some of which may be redundant. Pilot studies are performed where some of the questions are eliminated by statistical factor analyses.

Development of a Questionnaire

There are international guidelines (Scientific Advisory Committee of the Medical Outcome Trust, 2002) for the development and validation of health outcome measure questionnaires. The guidelines describe a rigorous, three-stage, gold standard methodology. It briefly comprises of three stages. In the first stage, a pool of items is generated from interviews with patient interviews and experts, and a review of the literature. This results in the development of a conceptual model. In the second stage, the large pool of items is field tested by postal survey to select questions that showed the best scientific performance. Scales are also identified at this stage. In the third stage the measurement properties of the new measure are further tested by a further postal survey of an independent group of patients.

The first stage in the development of a questionnaire is item generation that usually encompass a number of domains. A comprehensive selection of questions is identified along with responses that cover all aspects of the disease. This is done through patient and clinician interviews and review of the literature. This is followed by item reduction following a field test of the questionnaire where the number of questions is reduced to a reasonable size by removing unnecessary and repetitive questions. This also relies on expert opinion and statistical analyses to determine the redundancy of a question, its endorsement frequency and factor analyses. Missing data is also assessed to identify any trends and determine the cause for it and questions may need to be rephrases or removed.

This is followed by pilot studies and psychometric analyses. This allows the performance and relevance of the questions and the questionnaire as a whole to be assessed. Questions are then be statistically analysed to assess their validity and reliability before they are eliminated or rephrased. Pilot studies allow a trial of the questionnaire using a sample population that the questionnaire would ultimately be targeted at. The completed questionnaires are then statistically analysed to assess the acceptability, validity, internal consistency, item total correlation, reliability, responsiveness, bias and range. These are discussed at the end of the chapter.

In general, if there is more than 5% missing data for a particular question, it should be rephrased or removed. The endorsement frequency i.e. the proportion of respondents who endorse a particular response category, is also important. The endorsement frequency should be between 20% and 80%. If the endorsement frequency is outside this range, it suggests that there is inadequate spread of response categories. If a response for a particular question is chosen very often or not often enough, it suggests that the response has poor discriminatory power and that it is redundant and can be excluded.

In general there are two easy ways of analysing a pilot questionnaire. Item analysis is often used in pilot studies to decide if a question or response should be retained or deleted. High endorsement of a response option suggests poor discriminatory power and should be deleted. An alternative method is to use the Cronbach's alpha. This is used to show that the questionnaire measures a single construct and that questions can be combined to form a summary score. Cronbach's alpha coefficients for summary scores should be greater 0.70. A lower value suggests that the questions in the questionnaire are poorly grouped. It is important that individual questions measure distinct but related constructs. Item–total correlations for individual questions should have a value of greater than 0.30, and questions that have a value of less than 0.30 are assumed not to add to the value of the questionnaire and should be excluded.

However, despite the above analyses, it is important to bear in mind the original questionnaire and the theoretical domains, as these may sometimes overrule any poor statistical performance. Pilot studies are performed that aim to identify any potential problems with questionnaires so that they could be dealt with before the formal use of a questionnaire. Pilot studies can identify questions frequently omitted and look at the cause that may be inappropriate wording of a question. Pilot studies also allow the refining of words and content. Often open-ended questions are introduced only in pilot studies so further information and feedback from the questionnaire could be obtained.

Presentation of the Questionnaire

The way a questionnaire is presented is vital. A well structured questionnaire following a logical order that is easy to follow will result in a high response rate and have fewer omissions. It is important that there are clear explanations to the patients, often in the form of an accompanying letter, detailing the purpose of the questionnaire, why the patient has been asked to complete the questionnaire, and clear instructions on how to complete the questionnaire.

If open-ended questions are being used, it is important that there is enough space available for a response. It is important that the questionnaire is well-laid out, uses polite language and the text is readable. The order of the questions is also important and any optional questions should be included at the end of the questionnaires. Controversial and emotive questions should ideally be placed towards the end of the questionnaire. It is also worth arranging the questions with a mixture of positively and negatively worded questions to minimise acquiescent response bias. Although many of these statements are common sense, they can easily be overlooked in the difficult technicalities of developing the questionnaire.

The Ideal Patient-Completed Questionnaire

The ideal patient-completed questionnaire for outcome assessment of the hand, or indeed any outcome assessment, does not exist. The ideal questionnaire should enable the patient to convey the relevant information, and for the clinician to satisfactorily use that information. For this to happen, both the patient and the clinician need to be thought of when designing a questionnaire.

The questionnaire, as it is to be completed by the patient, should avoid technical terms as these may not be understood, or worse, misunderstood by the patient. They should avoid ambiguity and bias, and use simple short phrases. It is important to avoid 'double barrelled' questions, and 'double negative' questions. By making the questionnaire more acceptable to the patient, there should be a higher response rate and fewer omissions in the questionnaires.

It is also important that any questionnaire puts minimum burden on the rater or respondent in terms of time and effort to ensure optimal compliance. It should not place any financial burden on the respondent and postage should be paid for by the physician or researcher. It is also important that any questionnaire puts minimum administrative burden on the physician or researcher in terms of extracting information from the questionnaire, inputting data on a database and calculating the score.

Statistical Analyses of Questionnaires

With an increasing focus on patient reported regional outcome measures, many measures are now available. This makes the appropriate selection of an outcome measure difficult and emphasises the need for a greater understanding of how these measures should be analyses. The statistical analyses of regional outcome measures are guided by evidence of their validity, reliability, responsiveness, bias and practical considerations. These properties however are not fixed and the process of statistically analysing a questionnaire to determine whether or not it is appropriate in a particular setting and with a particular population is an ongoing process. These analyses may result in a refined regional outcome measure for a different settings or populations to those that the original regional outcome measure was developed for. These statistical features are all discussed below.

Validity

Many questionnaires are referred in the literature as 'validated instruments'. The concept of a validated instrument implies an inaccurate dichotomy that either the instrument is valid or it is not. A questionnaire's score will reflect the underlying construct more accurately or less accurately but never perfectly.

A questionnaire is considered valid if it does what it is supposed to. It is important to point out that a questionnaire's validity needs to be specified for a particular clinical situation. The M2 DASH questionnaire e.g. has been validated for hand injuries but not for shoulder dislocations or carpal tunnel syndromes. Each study thus provides evidence of the validity of a questionnaire for a particular clinical scenario, and a more complete picture of the validity of the questionnaire emerges as further studies are performed validating the questionnaire in different clinical scenarios. The validity of a questionnaire could be assessed by looking at the content, construct or criterion validity. The validity of a questionnaire is further supported by its responsiveness or ability to detect clinically significant changes over time.

1. Content validity

The content or face validity of a questionnaire is determined qualitatively by analysing the questions within the questionnaire to determine if they adequately cover relevant aspects that the questionnaire intends to assess. This could be done in many ways. It could be done by interviewing patients, interviewing experts or both. Historically this has been done by relying on experts but more recently there has been a greater appreciation of the need to include patients in this process. It could also be done by analysing the literature. Further information on the content validity of the questionnaire could be ascertained by performing the pilot study and the use of open-ended questions. This alone however is not sufficient to validate a questionnaire.

2. Construct validity

The construct or predictive validity of a questionnaire is assessed by assessing whether the scores obtained from the questionnaire are consistent with those expected or predicted given the clinical situation.

Statistical analyses of construct validity can be expressed in correlation coefficients, and generally involves looking at convergent or divergent validity. Convergent or concurrent, and divergent validity are demonstrated by correlating with similar and dissimilar measures. Depending on the type of validity that is studied, the value can vary. Construct validity is assessed by testing specific predefined hypotheses about expected correlations or differences in questionnaire scores between groups. If at least 75% of the scores are in accordance with the hypothesis, the construct of the questionnaire is considered valid.

3. Criterion validity

The criterion validity of a questionnaire is assessed by comparing the scores obtained by using the questionnaire with a 'gold standard' measure. This way of assessing the validity of a questionnaire is not applicable in many situations as a 'gold standard' does not exist; if it had, it would have been used as the outcome measure rather than the questionnaire in question. Although measurement of the grip strength in hand disorders is considered the gold standard for assessing validity by some (Sharma & Dias, 2000), others have shown that it performs variably depending on the pathology (Atroshi et al, 1999).

Convergent or concurrent, and divergent validity are demonstrated by correlating with similar and dissimilar measures. Correlation with other proven outcome measures is done using convergent validity. Evidence that the questionnaire is correlated with other questionnaires of similar constructs is assessed on the basis of correlations between the questionnaires. A value of 0.30-0.70 suggests moderate correlation. If the correlation with the criterion standard is greater than 0.70, the questionnaire is deemed to have good criterion validity.

Reliability

Reliability is concerned with the reproducibility of an instrument and is determined by the degree to which the instrument is free from random error. Questionnaires with low reliability only allow the detection of large group differences for a given sample size. This is estimated by examining the extent to which similar scores can be obtained with multiple replications of items, occasions and raters. The reliability can be assessed in different ways, each taking into account the replication of items, occasions and raters.

1. Internal consistency

The internal consistency or reliability of the items that make up the domain and questionnaire is tested by ensuring that all questions within the domain and questionnaire are relevant to that domain and questionnaire and are inter-correlated or internally consistent. This however is only applicable when there is more than one question to assess each domain.

In most questionnaires there are predetermined domains e.g. pain, function etc, and one or more questions for each domain. Many questionnaires have more than one question for each domain as it allows a more thorough assessment of each domain. Symptoms like pain and function are complex and multifaceted, and one question alone is generally insufficient to satisfactorily assess them. It is however important that all questions within the domain are relevant to that domain and are internally consistent. This is assessed by performing statistical analyses. This can be done using Cronbach's alpha statistic or the corrected item-total correlation.

The Cronbach's alpha gives an idea of the correlation of individual domain questions with all domain questions, and all questionnaire questions using inter-item correlations. A Cronbach's alpha gives a value between 0 and 1, and a value of < 0.70 suggests that the questions in the domain or the questionnaire are poorly grouped. Values > 0.70 suggest good internal consistency. A high Cronbach's alpha however, as seen with the DASH questionnaire, suggests some redundancy of the domain questions. This issue was one of the reasons that lead to the creation of the M2 DASH questionnaire, but formal statistical analyses on its internal reliability are yet to be performed.

Another way to assess internal consistency is using the corrected item-total correlation. The item-total correlation is the correlation between a question and the domain or the questionnaire. The corrected item-total correlation is the correlation between a question and the domain or the questionnaire corrected by removing the score for the question being analysed. Any question with a corrected item-total correlation of < 0.03 should be removed as it does not have significant correlation with other questions of the domain or the questionnaire. A high corrected item-total correlation of > 0.08 suggests that there is repetition in the questionnaire. Inter-item correlation values should be between 0.3 and 0.7.

Other statistical measures include the internal consistency coefficient. The kappa coefficients have also been reported as an estimate of reliability. It examines the proportion of responses in agreement at different measurement points. Kappa values of < 0.40 are poor, 0.40-0.59 are fair, 0.60-0.74 are good, and > 0.74 are excellent.

2. Test-retest reliability

The test-retest reliability or reproducibility of a questionnaire can be assessed by completing the questionnaire at two different instances and ensuring that the score does not change. It is however important to ensure that during the period between completing the two questionnaires, no significant clinical differences have taken place. Repeated measurements under constant clinical conditions should yield consistent and reproducible values. The period between test and retest is important. A significantly short period may result in recall of answers artificially increasing reliability. A significantly long period may result in an actual change in health. One way of getting round this problem is by using health transition questions that ask patients about any change in health between the test and retest, and only patients with no change in health are included in the analyses.

Reliability is established by calculating an interclass correlation coefficient for continuous measures. This is used to identify a group shift over time. This is done by dividing the variation in the population (inter-individual variation) by the total variation, which is the inter-individual variation plus the intra-individual variation (measurement error), expressed as a ratio between 0 and 1. For ordinal data, the weighted Cohen k coefficient should be used. For group comparisons, a value of 0.70 or higher is considered acceptable. More rigorous values are needed for individual comparisons, and a value of 0.90 or higher is considered acceptable.

The Pearson correlation may also be used and should be greater than 0.70 between test and retest questionnaire scores. This correlation however does not take systematic differences into account

3. Inter-rater reliability

The inter-rater reliability or reproducibility of a questionnaire can be assessed by two different raters completing the questionnaire in identical clinical scenarios and ensuring that the scores are similar. It is however important to ensure that the two raters experience identical clinical scenarios when completing the questionnaires. Measurements by different raters under constant clinical conditions should yield consistent and reproducible values.

It should be remembered that the reliability of a questionnaire is not intrinsic and can depend on the population studied. It is therefore important that the questionnaires, when moved for use to a different population group, is analysed again to ensure it remains statistically robust.

Responsiveness

A questionnaire is responsive if the score changes reflecting the change in the clinical situation. This is especially relevant as it allows a comparison between scores before and after an intervention. It is also relevant where it needs to be determined how long after an intervention the patients return to a certain level of activity. The responsiveness of a questionnaire is a relative property. In outcome studies, the DASH questionnaire has been shown to be less responsive than a disease-specific instrument following distal radial fractures (MacDermid et al, 2000) but equally responsive to the Carpal Tunnel Syndrome Evaluation Instrument when looking at carpal tunnel syndrome (Beaton et al, 2001).

Responsiveness is assessed by examining scores before and after a clinically significant change. There are two main approaches to analysing the responsiveness of questionnaires; distribution based approach and anchor based approach. Distribution based approaches relate changes in questionnaire scores to variability and use the change in mean score in the numerator, but with different denominators. The effect size (ES) is calculated by dividing the mean change in scores by the standard deviation of the baseline scores. A value of 0.50-0.80 suggests moderate to large effect sizes. The standardised response mean (SRM) is calculated by dividing the mean change in scores by the standard deviation of the score differences. Both the ES and the SRM are common measures of responsiveness. Positive values suggest improvements in score. An ES of 0.80 or more is considered as large, 0.50 or more is considered as moderate, and less than 0.50 is considered as small. The ES and SRM values can be compared with a comparable outcome measures to using the modified jack-knife test to analyse responsiveness. The two questionnaires should however measure the same domain or construct within the same patient group. Bonferroni correction is required if multiple paired testing is performed.

The ES and SRM may however be affected by the natural variance in the baseline condition and by the measurement error. The modified standardised response mean (MSRM), or responsiveness index, addresses the inherent natural variance that may be present in patients who report no changes to their health and the non specific change in score by only using the standard deviation of change in patients who report themselves as being stable. This would allow the detection of clinically important changes above the nonspecific change that is incorporated in the MSRM.

It is argued that the statistical measures of responsiveness described above are limited and patients' views on the importance of the change should determine the analyses. Anchor based approaches analyse the relationship between the changes in scores and a predetermined external variable e.g. the patient's perception of a change, to determine a Minimal Important Difference (MID).

Range

It is important that measurements reflect true changes in the clinical situation without ceiling or floor effects. A ceiling effect occurs when a large cluster of patient scores are located at the top end of the questionnaire scale, whereas a floor effect occurs when a large cluster of scores are located at the bottom end of a scale. These occur due to the skewing of the score distribution and limit the ability to detect changes in the measurements that may otherwise be clinically significant. Ceiling effects result in a type II error when testing hypotheses and fail to show improvements in clinical situation

Questionnaires that are attempting to deal with the ceiling and floor effect include computerised questionnaires that rely on the item response theory (Wood-Dauphinee, 1999). The computerised programme allows the adaptive testing of the questionnaire tailored to the patient and each response determines the subsequent question.

Bias

In all the above questionnaires there are predetermined domains e.g. pain, function etc, and one or more questions for each domain. Many questionnaires have more than one question for each domain as it allows a more thorough assessment of each domain. Symptoms like pain and function are complex and multifaceted, and one question alone is generally insufficient to satisfactorily assess them. A number of questions also allows a more thorough assessment of the domain and reduce the chances of bias due to a single answer.

The layout of the questionnaire, the type of question, the language used and the order of the questions may all bias response. Controversial and emotive questions should ideally be placed towards the end of the questionnaire. It is also worth arranging the questions with a mixture of positively and negatively worded questions to minimise acquiescent response bias.

Bias is determined by using discriminant validity. Convergent or concurrent, and divergent validity are demonstrated by correlating with similar and dissimilar measures. Evidence that a questionnaire is not correlated with different variables is assessed on the basis of correlations with age, sex etc giving a low correlations of less than 0.30.

Practical Considerations

Ideally the questionnaire should enable the patient to convey the relevant information, and for the clinician to satisfactorily use that information. The questionnaire needs to be practical in clinical practice. This means it should be acceptable, feasible and appropriate. There are many ways in which a questionnaire could be made more acceptable, feasible and appropriate for the patient and the clinician; very often the two go hand in hand. The acceptability of a questionnaire relates to the ability and willingness of the patient and the clinicians to use a questionnaire. Feasibility relates to the time, resources and effort required to complete, collect, process, score and analyse a questionnaire. Appropriateness relates to how appropriate a particular questionnaire is for the intended purpose.

1. Acceptability

Acceptability determines the ability and willingness of patients to complete a questionnaire and the clinicians to use it. Although it is difficult to evaluate the acceptability of a questionnaire directly, it can be determined indirectly by response rates and completion. Patients are unlikely to answer questions that they perceive as irrelevant or inappropriate, or where the response options are limited. Patients with disease and injury of the hand may experience problems with writing and may not prefer completing lengthy responses to open questions. The way a questionnaire is presented is important and a well structured questionnaire following a logical order that is easy to follow will result in a high response rate and have fewer omissions. Other important factors that are commonly overlooked are the first language of the patient, the layout of the questionnaire and the size and style of font used. For clinicians, the acceptability of a questionnaire does depend on the general perception of the questionnaire and its acceptability by the profession as a whole. The layout and the scoring method also affect the acceptability of a questionnaire to the clinicians. It should also be remembered that the questionnaires are very often used by allied healthcare disciplines and not only surgeons.

During the questionnaire development stages, the questionnaire should be analysed by patient and clinician groups and any perceived problems regarding the content, format and layout ironed out at an early stage.

2. Feasibility

The feasibility of a questionnaire relates to the time, resources and effort required to complete, collect, process, score and analyse a questionnaire. This has implications on both the patient and the clinician, and is one of the main reasons that questionnaires are not used more routinely. The questionnaires discussed in this chapter are freely available but others such as the SF-36 have copyright and associated cost issues.

It is also important that any questionnaire puts minimum burden on the patient in terms of time and effort to ensure optimal compliance. It should not place any financial burden on the respondent and postage for postal surveys should be paid for by the clinician. It is also important that any questionnaire puts minimum administrative burden on the physician or researcher in terms of extracting information from the questionnaire, inputting data on a database and calculating the score.

3. Appropriateness

With the increasing use of a number of questionnaires as regional outcome measures, there is a need to identify the most appropriate questionnaire relevant to any clinical setting and patient population. This chapter looks at how questionnaires are designed and also look at the statistical analyses of questionnaires to determine their validity and reliability. This information should enable the readers to critically analyse various questionnaires and have a better idea regarding the statistical robustness of them.

Regional Outcome Measures in Common Use

With an increasing number of treatment modalities becoming available, and with the emphasis on evidence-based practice, there is an ever-increasing use of regional outcome measures used in the assessment of patients to identify the optimal treatment modality. These questionnaires are useful as they do not provide limited information about one modality e.g. pain or function, but rather provide a single measure for multiple modalities. It also encompasses a range of symptoms including the physical, social and psychological. It is important that hand surgeons and other disciplines involved with the care of patients with hand injury and disease have an understanding of the commonly used hand questionnaires.

Disabilities of the Arm Shoulder and Hand Questionnaire

The DASH questionnaire was developed for use in North America (Beaton et al, 2001) but translated versions have been validated in a number of languages including French and Japanese (Imaeda et al, 2005), Spanish (Hervás et al, 2006) and German (Westphal, 2007).

The Disability of the Arm, Shoulder and Hand (DASH) questionnaire (Hudak et al., 1996) is probably the most commonly used patient-completed regional outcome measure used for the hand (Khan et al, 2004; Khan & Fahmy, 2006). The main developmental objective was to develop a patient-reported regional outcome measure which considers the upper limb as a single functional unit allowing greater uniformity. The DASH questionnaire measures symptoms and functional status in patients with disorders of the upper limb. It was originally designed and validated as a measure of disability in patients with upper limb disorders. The DASH questionnaire is used in orthopaedics, rheumatology and neurology to assess self-reported patient outcome (Jupiter & Ring, 2002; McKee et al, 2003).

Development of the DASH Questionnaire

During the development of the questionnaire, 13 scales and 821 items used in measuring the outcomes of various upper limb conditions were chosen after an extensive literature review. Staged item reduction was performed based on expert opinion to 177 items, based on content experts to 75 items, and following pilot testing to 30 items. This includes 21 physical function items, 6 symptom items and 3 social function items. The six domains assessed in the DASH questionnaire are daily activities, symptoms, social function, work function, sleep and confidence. There are also two optional modules, the high performance sports module and the work module.

The score out of 100 is calculated from the questionnaire after the patient answers 30 questions, evaluating symptoms and physical function, choosing one of five responses from a five-point Likert scale. The final score is calculated using the formula below

DASH Score= ((Average Response per Question Answered) - 1) X 25

The DASH questionnaire allows for the omission of up to three questions. It is a time-consuming outcome measure and takes the patient 10 to 15 minutes to complete, and the clinician 5 minutes to calculate the final score.

Statistical Analyses

In 2001, Beaton et al studied 200 patients with either, wrist and hand or shoulder problems to determine the validity, test-retest reliability and responsiveness of the DASH questionnaire. Correlations or t-tests between the DASH and the other measures were used to assess construct validity. Beaton et al found the DASH questionnaire to correlate well with other measures including the Brigham questionnaire, the Shoulder Pain and Disability Index (SPADI) and other markers of pain and function ($r > 0.69$). Eighty-six patients completed a further questionnaire after three to five days and test-retest reliability was determined by intra-class correlation coefficient (ICC=0.96). Responsiveness was determined using the standardised response means and correlations between change in DASH questionnaire score and change in scores of other measures, and showed that the responsiveness of the DASH was either comparable with or better than the joint-specific measures. The DASH was shown to be responsive with changes found to correlate well with changes in the patient's condition. The standardised response mean of 0.74 for the DASH questionnaire was comparable to 0.76 for joint specific outcome measures e.g. the Brigham score.

The DASH questionnaire has a good correlation with the International Classification of Functioning, Disability and Health (Drummond et al, 2007). The DASH questionnaire has also been shown to have a good correlation with radiological and objective physical results (Wilcke et al, 2007). The DASH questionnaire showed convergent validity through a correlation with other joint specific instruments, such as the Brigham Carpal Tunnel Questionnaire (0.73) and the Shoulder Pain and Disability Index (0.72). It has shown validity and responsiveness in both proximal and distal disorders suggesting usefulness in all upper limb disorders (Beaton et al, 2001). The DASH questionnaire showed a weaker correlation with severity of pain in the wrist joint (0.67) suggesting that it was less valid for use in patients with wrist injuries or disease.

The DASH questionnaire has been shown to be reliable with a Cronbach's alpha of 0.90-0.97 in a number of studies suggesting good internal consistency (Van de Ven-Stevens et al, 2009). The test–retest reliability was assessed in 86 patients who were asked to complete the questionnaire at baseline and then three to five days later. The Pearson correlation between the baseline and retest scores was 0.96 suggesting excellent reproducibility. In other studies the DASH questionnaire showed an interclass correlation coefficient of 0.95 and 0.96 for a total population of 88 and 56 patients respectively, and a Pearson correlation coefficient of 0.98 for the total DASH scores of the initial assessment and the reassessment in 50 patients (Van de Ven-Stevens et al, 2009).

Disadvantages of the DASH Questionnaire

It was originally developed as a regional outcome measure specific for the upper limb but recent studies showed that patients with lower limb disability had DASH scores higher than normal control subjects (Dowrick et al, 2006; Khan et al, 2008). This suggests that the questionnaire does not exclusively measure disability associated with disorders of the upper limb. This means that in studies looking at DASH scores where there were injuries to both upper and lower limbs, and in studies of polyarthropathies, the DASH scores need to be interpreted with caution.

A study investigating the construct validity of the DASH questionnaire was performed to determine whether the questionnaire measures disability solely attributed to the upper limb (Khan et al, 2008). One hundred and ninety two patients completed the DASH questionnaire, including 79 patients with upper limb injuries, 61 patients with lower limb injuries and 52 control subjects. The DASH scores were calculated and comparisons of the scores between the three groups were made using the Kruskal-Wallis test. Pairwise comparisons between the groups were also made using the Mann-Whitney test. The mean DASH scores and standard deviations for the three groups were 54 (22) for the upper limb group, 16 (10) for the lower limb group, and 2 (3) for the control group, and the scores varied significantly between the three groups (Kruskal-Wallis: $p<0.001$). The mean score for the upper limb group were higher than the lower limb group (Mann-Whitney: $p<0.001$), and the mean score for the lower limb group was higher than the control group (Mann-Whitney: $p<0.001$) (Figure 1).

Patients with lower limb pathologies who completed the DASH questionnaire scored significantly higher than the control suggesting that the questions are not specific for the upper limb. This was because the DASH questionnaire includes questions that do not solely rely on the function of the upper limb e.g. 'ability to make a bed' or 'ability to manage transportation needs'. These questions thus address both lower and upper limb disability. Other questions in the DASH questionnaire do not involve the use of the lower limb function e.g. 'ability to turn a key' or 'ability to open a jar'.

Statistical analyses of the original DASH questionnaire has also showed a high internal consistency (Dias et al, 2008) suggesting redundancy in questions. The original DASH questionnaire also has other limitations. It is difficult to reproduce as it spans four pages, it is somewhat lengthy with 30 questions, the completion of the optional modules is variable, and importantly it is not specific for the upper limb. These issues prompted the authors to create a modified shorter version, the M^2 DASH that is more specific for the upper limb.

Manchester-Modified Disabilities of the Arm Shoulder and Hand Questionnaire

There are many outcome measures described in literature but not many are specific to the hand. The Disabilities of Arm, Shoulder and Hand (DASH) questionnaire was developed as a region specific outcome measure for the upper limb. A recent study however has shown that the DASH questionnaire is not specific for the upper limb and also measures disability in the lower limb (Khan et al, 2008). A modified DASH score was created with fewer questions that can discriminate clearly between disabilities due to problems at the upper limb, and was more specific to the upper limb (Khan et al, 2008). The M^2 DASH questionnaire is not limited by lower limb pathologies and is more sensitive and specific for the upper limb. In isolated upper limb injuries the M^2 DASH questionnaire shows a good correlation with the original DASH questionnaire (Khan et al, 2008).This questionnaire could satisfactorily be used in patients with both upper and lower limb disability, and only measure the disability in the upper limb.

One hundred and ninety two patients completed the DASH questionnaire, including 79 patients with upper limb injuries, 61 patients with lower limb injuries and 52 control subjects. The DASH scores were calculated and showed significant differences between the upper injury group, the lower injury group and the control group. The scores of the lower injury group were significantly higher than the control group suggesting that the DASH score measures disability attributed to the lower limb. Using the frequency tables and bar charts for the scores for each group for each question, questions that the lower limb injury group scored highly on were identified and eliminated, resulting in the revised Manchester-Modified or M^2 DASH questionnaire containing questions specific to the upper limb (Table 1). The M^2 DASH questionnaire thus included questions 1-4, 6, 13-17, 21-23 and 26-30 from the original questionnaire and is shown in Figure 1. The revised questionnaire retains at least half the number of questions from each of the six domains described in the original DASH questionnaire. It allows the omission of up to two questions and the score is calculated just like the original questionnaire by adding up the total scores from all answered questions, dividing it by the number of answered questions, subtracting 1 and multiplying by 25.

Manchester-Modified Disability of the Arm, Shoulder and Hand (M^2 DASH) questionnaire

Patient's Name/ Reference.. **Date**..................................

Clinician's Name/ Reference..

INSTRUCTIONS FOR PATIENT: This questionnaire asks about your symptoms as well as you ability to perform certain activities. Please answer every question, based on your condition in the last week. If you did not have the opportunity to perform an activity in the past week, please make your best estimate on which response would be the most accurate. It doesn't matter which hand or arm you use to perform the activity; please answer based on you ability regardless of how you perform the task.

Please rate your ability to do the following activities in the last week.	No difficulty	Mild difficulty	Moderate difficulty	Severe difficulty	Unable
1. Open a tight or new jar	1	2	3	4	5
2. Write	1	2	3	4	5
3. Turn a key	1	2	3	4	5
4. Prepare a meal	1	2	3	4	5
5. Place an object on a shelf above your head	1	2	3	4	5
6. Wash or blow dry your hair	1	2	3	4	5
7. Wash your back	1	2	3	4	5
8. Put on a pullover sweater	1	2	3	4	5
9. Use a knife to cut food	1	2	3	4	5
10. Recreational activities which require little effort (eg cardplaying, knitting, etc)	1	2	3	4	5
11. Sexual activities	1	2	3	4	5
	Not at all	Slightly	Moderately	Quite a bit	Extremely
12. During the past week, to what extent has your arm, shoulder or hand problem interfered with your normal social activities with family, friends, neighbours or groups?	1	2	3	4	5
	Not limited at all	Slightly limited	Moderately limited	Very limited	Unable
13. During the past week, were you limited in your work or other regular daily activities as a result of your arm, shoulder or hand problem?	1	2	3	4	5
14. Tingling (pins and needles) in your arm, shoulder or hand	1	2	3	4	5
15. Weakness in your arm, shoulder or hand	1	2	3	4	5
16. Stiffness in your arm, shoulder or hand	1	2	3	4	5
	No difficulty	Mild difficulty	Moderate difficulty	Severe difficulty	So much difficulty I can't sleep
17. During the past week, how much difficulty have you had sleeping because of the pain in your arm, shoulder or hand?	1	2	3	4	5
	Strongly disagree	Disagree	Neither agree or disagree	Agree	Strongly agree
18. I feel less capable, less confident or less useful because of my arm, shoulder or hand problem	1	2	3	4	5

Thank you very much for completing all the questions in this questionnaire.

INSTRUCTIONS FOR CLINICIAN: The questionnaire can only be used if at least 16 out of the 18 questions have been answered. Using the formula below, you get a score out of 100.

$$\left(\left(\frac{\text{SUM OF TOTAL SCORE}}{\text{NUMBER OF QUESTIONS ANSWERED}}\right) \text{SUBTRACT 1}\right) \text{MULTIPLY BY 25} = \ldots\ldots\ldots\ldots$$

Reference: Khan WS, Jain R, Dillon B, Clarke L, Fehily M, Ravenscroft M (2008). Hand; 3(3): 240-244.

Figure 1. M2 DASH questionnaire in the one-page format including the instructions for patients and clinicians, and the equation for score calculation.

Table 1. The original DASH, QuickDASH and M^2 DASH questionnaires

Please rate your ability to do the following activities in the last week.	No difficulty	Mild difficulty	Moderate difficulty	Severe difficulty	Unable
1. Open a tight or new jar	1	2	3	4	5
2. Write	1	2	3	4	5
3. Turn a key	1	2	3	4	5
4. Prepare a meal	1	2	3	4	5
5. Push open a heavy door	1	2	3	4	5
6. Place an object on a shelf above your head	1	2	3	4	5
7. Do heavy household chores (eg wash walls, wash floors)	1	2	3	4	5
8. Garden or do yard work	1	2	3	4	5
9. Make a bed	1	2	3	4	5
10. Carry a shopping bag or briefcase	1	2	3	4	5
11. Carry a heavy object (over 10 lbs)	1	2	3	4	5
12. Change a lightbulb overhead	1	2	3	4	5
13. Wash or blow dry your hair	1	2	3	4	5
14. Wash your back	1	2	3	4	5
15. Put on a pullover sweater	1	2	3	4	5
16. Use a knife to cut food	1	2	3	4	5
17. Recreational activities which require little effort (eg cardplaying, knitting, etc)	1	2	3	4	5
18. Recreational activities in which you take some force or impact through your arm, shoulder or hand (eg golf, hammering, tennis, etc)	1	2	3	4	5

Table 1. (Continued)

Please rate your ability to do the following activities in the last week.	No difficulty	Mild difficulty	Moderate difficulty	Severe difficulty	Unable
19. Recreational activities in which you move your arm freely (eg playing frisbee, badminton, etc)	1	2	3	4	5
20. Manage transportation needs (getting from one place to another)	1	2	3	4	5
21. Sexual activities	1	2	3	4	5
	Not at all	Slightly	Moderately	Quite a bit	Extremely
22. During the past week, to what extent has your arm, shoulder or hand problem interfered with your normal social activities with family, friends, or groups?	1	2	3	4	5
	Not limited at all	Slightly limited	Moderately limited	Very limited	Unable
23. During the past week, were you limited in your work or other regular daily activities as a result of your arm, shoulder or hand problem?	1	2	3	4	5
24. Arm, shoulder or hand pain	1	2	3	4	5
25. Arm, shoulder or hand pain when you performed any specific activity	1	2	3	4	5

Table 1. (Continued)

Please rate your ability to do the following activities in the last week.	No difficulty	Mild difficulty	Moderate difficulty	Severe difficulty	Unable
25. Arm, shoulder or hand pain when you performed any specific activity	1	2	3	4	5
26. Tingling (pins and needles) in your arm, shoulder or hand	1	2	3	4	5
27. Weakness in your arm, shoulder or hand	1	2	3	4	5
28. Stiffness in your arm, shoulder or hand	1	2	3	4	5
	No difficulty	Mild difficulty	Moderate difficulty	Severe difficulty	So much difficulty I can't sleep
29. During the past week, how much difficulty have you had sleeping because of the pain in your arm, shoulder or hand?	1	2	3	4	5
	Strongly disagree	Disagree	Neither agree or disagree	Agree	Strongly agree
30. I feel less capable, less confident or less useful because of my arm, shoulder or hand problem	1	2	3	4	5

The table shows the 30 questions that form the original DASH questionnaire. The QuickDASH questions are highlighted in italics and the M^2 DASH questions are highlighted in bold. The score is calculated by adding up the total scores for each answered question, dividing it by the number of answered questions, subtracting 1 and multiplying by 25. This applies to all three questionnaires and gives a score out of 100 (Khan et al, 2008).

Comparison of the M^2 DASH scores between the three groups was also made using the Kruskal-Wallis test, followed by pair-wise comparisons between the groups using the Mann-Whitney test. The mean M^2 DASH scores and standard deviations for the three groups were 51 (23) for the upper limb group, 9 (9) for the lower limb group, and 2 (2) for the control group. The M^2 DASH scores varied significantly between the three groups (Kruskal-Wallis: $p<0.001$). Pair-wise comparisons between the upper and lower limb groups (Mann-Whitney: $p<0.001$), and between the upper limb and control groups (Mann-Whitney: $p<0.001$) showed statistically significant differences. Importantly, no significant difference was seen between the lower limb group and the control group (Mann-Whitney: $p>0.05$) when using the M^2 DASH scores unlike the DASH scores (Figure 2). Using chi-square tests, only question 10 ($p>0.05$) and question 20 ($p>0.05$) showed no evidence of a difference between the upper limb and lower limb group, suggesting that they were not specific for the upper limb group. These two questions were not in the M^2 DASH questionnaire. The M^2 DASH questionnaire score was then calculated for the group of patients with upper limb injury and a correlation study performed with the original DASH questionnaire score to assess the validity of the modified questionnaire. This showed a high correlation (Spearman's correlation coefficient, $r=0.98$, $p<0.001$) confirming that the ranking of the upper limb patients is similar in the two questionnaires.

The authors of the study developed the M^2 DASH after excluding questions that were not specific to the upper limb. The purpose of developing the M^2 DASH questionnaire was to devise a questionnaire that is more specific for upper limb injuries and disease.

The M^2 DASH questionnaire was devised by excluding twelve questions from the DASH questionnaire that were not specific for the upper limb including 'ability to carry a shopping bag or briefcase' and 'ability to manage transportation needs'. In the modified questionnaire, at least half the questions from the original questionnaire's six domains remain. The questionnaire allows for the omission of up to two questions and the score is adjusted to accommodate for this. The study describing the M^2 DASH questionnaire showed a significant correlation between the scores obtained using the original and revised questionnaires in the group with upper limb injury also suggesting that the revised questionnaire is valid.

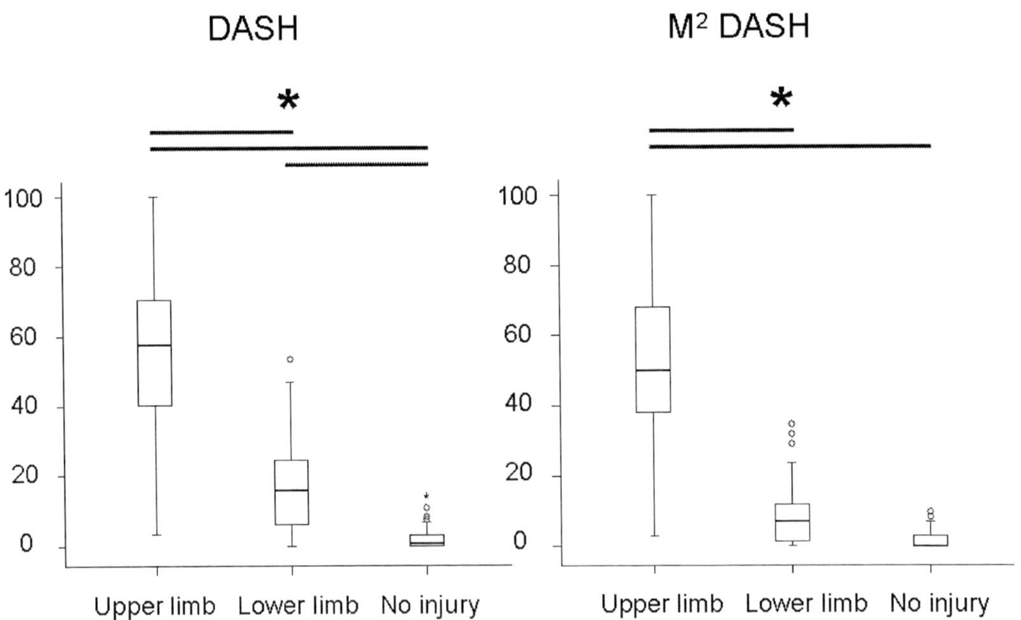

Figure 2. The dataset showing the distribution of DASH scores obtained using (a) the original DASH questionnaire and (b) the revised DASH questionnaire, for the upper limb injury group, lower limb injury group and the control group. The results show that the lower limb group scores are lower with the revised questionnaire (Khan et al, 2008).

The M^2 DASH questionnaire has construct validity as the questionnaire retains at least half of the questions from each of the six domains of the original DASH questionnaire (Khan et al, 2008). The M^2 DASH questionnaire includes some questions that do not form part of the routine objective assessments of the hand, suggesting good content or face validity.

As the only previous assessment of the validity of the M^2 DASH questionnaire was by comparison with the original DASH questionnaire from which the M^2 DASH scores had been extrapolated, a more thorough investigation was needed._It is important to determine the validity, reliability, responsiveness and bias of the newly created M2 DASH questionnaire. The validity establishes whether the outcome measure actually measures what it has been designed to. An outcome tool is reliable if the same score is obtained at different time points after the clinical condition has stabilised. The responsiveness is the ability to detect clinically important changes at different intervals. Bias can occur when variables assumed to be independent, such as age and gender, affect scores. The Patient Evaluation Measure (PEM) questionnaire was developed in the UK in 1995 (Macey et al, 1995), and the Michigan Hand Outcome (MHO) questionnaire was developed in the USA in 1998 (Chung et al, 1998). Both questionnaires are patient-completed region-specific outcome measures commonly used for hand injuries. In a more recent study we assessed the validity, reliability, responsiveness and bias of the M^2 DASH questionnaire for hand injuries using completed M^2 DASH, PEM and MHO questionnaires (Khan et al, in press).

Fifty nine patients with hand injuries who completed the M^2 DASH, PEM and MHO questionnaires at their first clinic visit, on discharge following their last visit, and at six months following discharge were studied. Patients were also asked to complete the M^2 DASH 12 months following discharge. Nine patients were lost to follow-up, six had a further injury or a recurrence of the previous injury, and four had inadequately completed questionnaires. Questionnaires from the remaining 40 patients with injuries to the hand were used to assess the validity, reliability, responsiveness and bias of the M^2 DASH questionnaire. The M^2 DASH, PEM and MHO scores were then calculated.

The validity of the M^2 DASH was assessed by determining how well the questionnaire score correlated with the PME and MHO scores. Using histograms it was determined that the scores were normally distributed, and Pearson correlations were used to compare the scores. Criterion validity testing showed strong correlations between the M^2 DASH scores and the PME and MHO scores suggesting that the M^2 DASH score measures what it is designed to and confirmed that the questionnaire is valid for injuries to the hand. The M^2 DASH scores showed highly significant positive correlations with the PEM and MHO scores at all three time points ($p<0.001$) as shown in Table 2. The magnitude of the correlation coefficient was slightly lower with the MHO scores than the PEM scores, and at six months following discharge than earlier.

The reliability was determined by performing test-retest analyses on the M^2 DASH scores at six and 12 months following discharge. Six months following discharge, as the patients had not sustained any further injury or sought further medical advice for the original injury, it was assumed that their condition had stabilised. There was a statistically significant correlation between the M^2 DASH scores six months and 12 months following discharge ($r=0.73$, $p<0.001$) suggesting good test-retest reproducibility and reliability.

Table 2. The correlations of PEM and MHO scores with the M² DASH scores.

Time of score	PEM score		MHO score	
	Correlation coefficent	p value	Correlation coefficent	P value
At presentation	0.96	<0.001	0.85	<0.001
At discharge	0.96	<0.001	0.88	<0.001
Six months following discharge	0.60	<0.001	0.54	<0.001

Responsiveness was determined by correlating the changes in the M² DASH score with changes in the PEM and MHO scores. This was done by calculating the effect size and the standardised response mean. The effect sizes were calculated by dividing the mean of change in the scores during the period from initial presentation to discharge, and from discharge to six months following discharge, by the standard deviation of the baseline score. The standardised response mean was calculated by dividing the mean of change in the scores between initial presentation and six months following discharge by the standard deviation of the change in score. The effect sizes for the M² DASH scores were 1.45 and 1.07 for the time periods between presentation and discharge, and between discharge and six months following discharge respectively as shown in Table 3. These values were greater than 0.8 suggesting that they were valuable. The effect sizes for the two periods were greater than those for the PME scores (1.26 and 0.96) and MHO scores (1.23 and 0.60). The effect size for the MHO scores between discharge and six months following discharge was less than 0.80 suggesting that they were not valuable. The standardised response means for the M² DASH, PME and MHO scores were 2.21, 1.80 and 1.50 respectively, suggesting that the M² DASH is a highly responsive scale. This study established that the M² DASH questionnaire is responsive to change compared with the PME and MHO questionnaires from initial presentation following injury through discharge from the fracture clinic and to 6 months following discharge.

Table 3: The effect sizes and standardised response means for the M² DASH, PME and MHO scores.

	M² DASH score	PEM score	MHO score
Effect size between presentation and discharge	1.45	1.26	1.23
Effect size between discharge and six month following discharge	1.07	0.96	0.6
Standardised response mean	2.21	1.80	1.50

The bias was investigated by performing correlation studies for assumed independent variables including age, gender, hand dominance, the side injured. Table 4 shows that there was no association between the M² DASH scores at presentation and 12 months following discharge, and gender, dominance and injury to dominant side confirming no bias. There was evidence of a weak association between age and the M² DASH score at presentation but the correlation coefficient was not large (r=0.37, p=0.02). The positive correlation implies that older patients have higher DASH scores when they present with hand injuries. There are two possible explanations for this. Either older patients sustain more severe hand injuries or sustain injuries of similar severity but suffer a greater disability as a result of the injury. Although the latter explanation is more likely, further work is needed to explore this in more detail. There was no correlation at 12 months following discharge (r=-0.09, p=0.57).

Table 4. The association between the M^2 DASH score and gender, dominance and injury to dominant side.

Association between M^2 DASH score and gender							
	Male			Female			
	N	Mean	SD	N	Mean	SD	p value
At presentation	24	52.3	18.7	16	47.9	23.8	0.52
12 months following discharge	24	4.8	2.7	16	5.4	2.5	0.49
Association between M^2 DASH score and dominance							
	Right			Left			
	N	Mean	SD	N	Mean	SD	p value
At presentation	31	51.9	20.8	9	45.8	20.8	0.44
12 months following discharge	31	5.2	2.7	9	4.4	2.2	0.45
Association between M^2 DASH score and injury to dominant side							
	Dominant injury			Non-dominant injury			
	N	Mean	SD	N	Mean	SD	p value
At presentation	26	48.2	21.2	14	54.9	19.8	0.34
12 months following discharge	26	4.9	2.6	14	5.2	2.6	0.74

Initial studies suggest that the M^2 DASH questionnaire is a robust region specific outcome measure. It is a valid and responsive questionnaire with test-retest reliability proven for hand injuries. Gender, handedness and side injured did not cause bias in the responses. There is a need for further studies looking beyond hand injuries before a more complete picture on the validity of the M^2 DASH for all upper limb pathologies could be drawn.

The M^2 DASH is an upper limb outcome assessment tool that is not pathology or region specific within the upper limb. It has a simple one-page layout and is easy to understand and complete for the patient. For the researcher, it is easy to enter into a database, and to calculate and analyse the score.

Patient Evaluation Measure Questionnaire

The Patient Evaluation Measure (PEM) questionnaire was developed in the United Kingdom in 1995 by Macey et al and assesses patient satisfaction with treatment, general hand functioning and activities of daily living. Unlike the DASH and MHO questionnaires, it has not formally been psychometrically evaluated.

There are only a few studies that have statistically analysed the questionnaire. Dias et al (2001) studied the reliability, validity, responsiveness and bias of the questionnaire (Table 5), and found it to be reliable, valid, responsive and free from bias. They studied 80 patients with acute scaphoid fractures at two, eight, twelve, twenty-six and fifty-two weeks following injury. The patients had a mean age of 29.7 years (SD 10.1 years). Patients with pre-existing wrist or hand disorders were excluded from the study. The patients were assessed at each visit where a history was taken and the patient examined. The patients were questioned about pain and swelling, the hand was examined for tenderness, range of wrist movements were measured using a goniometer, grip strength was measured using a dynamometer, and patients were asked to complete the PEM questionnaire.

The PEM questionnaire has a simple, uncluttered and easy to follow layout. Questions are short and simple, and are in a visual analogue form, and the patients only have to read the question, and not the description of the interval answers. The questions can be answered on a seven-interval visual analogue scale. The questionnaire is easy to enter into a database and to analyse. The questionnaire included three sections including a five question section assessing patients' view of treatment, and three question section assessing patients' overall assessment. There was an eleven question section assessing the hand health profile and included an added question on duration of pain that was absent in the original questionnaire. The PEM questionnaire score was calculated by adding the response to each question from sections two and three, and expressing the sum as a percentage of the maximum possible score.

The validity was assessed by determining how well responses to each question of the questionnaire and the total PEM questionnaire score, correlated with subjective and objective measures of function including pain, tenderness, swelling, wrist movements and grip strength. The study showed that the PEM was highly valid since it correlated well with other measures commonly used in the assessments of the function of the wrist and hand. Each individual question and the total PEM questionnaire score correlated well with the pain, tenderness, swelling, range of movement and grip strength. They established that the questions in the PEM questionnaire are highly internally consistent. The questions address different facets of the symptoms, function and cosmesis of the hand. The face validity of the questionnaire appears sound; it includes questions not usually included in the assessment of patients e.g. 'When I look at the appearance of my hand now, I feel: unconcerned. embarrassed and self-conscious' and 'Generally, when I think about my hand I feel: unconcerned. very upset'.

The reliability was assessed by measuring the internal consistency of the eleven questions in the hand health profile section and the three questions in the overall assessment section. They measured the correlation of each question with the others and generated Cronbach's alpha. The correlations of some of the questions e.g. 'When I try to use my hand for fiddly things, it is now: skilful......... clumsy', 'The grip in my hand is now: strong......... weak' and 'Generally, my hand is now: very satisfactory......... very unsatisfactory' with the rest of the scale was high at 0.83, 0.84 and 0.84, respectively. The correlations of some questions e.g. 'When I look at the appearance of my hand now, I feel: unconcerned......... embarrassed and self-conscious', 'Generally when I think about my hand I feel: unconcerned.......... very upset' and 'Generally, my treatment at the hospital has been: very satisfactory.......... very unsatisfactory' with the rest of the scale was particularly low at 0.36, 0.43 and 0.34 respectively.

The questionnaire was considered to be internally consistent if Cronbach's alpha was between 0.7 and 0.9. The Cronbach's alpha, calculating from these correlations was found to be 0.9, and suggested internal consistency. A very high internal consistency of >0.9 suggests that there is some redundancy with questions are measuring the same aspect twice. There was overall correlation across visits and for each visit. Cronbach's alpha at weeks 2, 8, 12, 26 and 52, were 0.874, 0.905, 0.939, 0.912 and 0.911 respectively. The overall value over time was 0.932 because of the added effect of the correlation due to changes in the group mean score over time. If a question disproportionately contributes to the internal consistency, then deleting it will result in a fall in Cronbach's alpha. If a question does not disproportionately contribute to the internal consistency, then deleting it will cause the Cronbach's alpha will rise. In the study, the Cronbach's alpha remained close to the 0.9, suggesting that each question contributed to the overall score and the PEM questionnaire is reliable. The degree of contribution of each question was studied by measuring the corrected Cronbach's alpha value after excluding that particular item.

To assess responsiveness, the changes between visits in the PEM questionnaire score and the pain, tenderness, swelling, wrist movement and grip strength were assessed. Changes in the PEM questionnaire score were correlated with changes in each of the other variables. Responsiveness was measured by calculating the effect size and by assessing the standardised response mean. Responsiveness was assessed by looking at the correlation between the variation in the questionnaire to changes in pain, tenderness, swelling, range of movement and grip strength. Pain and grip strength correlated significantly ($p < 0.001$) with changes in the PEM questionnaire score between the second and eighth weeks. Tenderness, range of movement and grip strength correlated significantly ($p < 0.03$) with changes in the PEM questionnaire score between the eighth and fifty second weeks. The effect size was calculated by dividing the mean of the change in the PEM questionnaire score between visits by the standard deviation of the baseline PEM questionnaire score. The effect size for the PEM questionnaire score was 1.12 and, as it was greater than 0.8, it was valuable. This effect size matched the effect sizes for swelling, tenderness, range of movement and grip strength at various stages between the second and fifty second weeks. The standardised response mean was calculated by dividing the mean of change in the PEM questionnaire score between visits at weeks 2 and 8 and between weeks 8 and 52 by the standard deviation of the change in PEM questionnaire score. The standardised response mean was 1.46 and 1.47 between visits at weeks 2 and 8 and between weeks 8 and 52 respectively. These assessments suggested that the PEM questionnaire is highly responsive.

Bias was studied by measuring the variance of each PEM question and the PEM questionnaire score for assumed independent variables including gender, hand dominance, the side injured and injuries to the dominant hand. Age bias was studied by correlating age with the PEM questionnaire score. The effects of subject factors were tested in a repeated measures analysis of variance, incorporating a fixed effect for the visit and a random effect for the subject. The study showed no item bias for gender, dominance and side injured. There was significant correlation with age at 0.01, suggesting that older patients had a lower PEM questionnaire score. This finding may be due to a poorer outcome in older individuals, and this was supported by a regression analysis of age and grip strength (p= 0.002).

The study concluded that the PEM is internally consistent, highly valid and responsive. They showed that gender, age, handedness and side injured did not cause bias in the responses to the questions. One potential flaw in the methodology of this study was that at each visit, the patients were told what their questionnaire answers had been at their previous visit. This could have determined the subsequent responses but nevertheless was needed to avoid bias and would have improved the consistency for this visual analogue scale response.

In 2005, Hobby et al studied the validity of the PEM questionnaire as an outcome measure in 24 patients with carpal tunnel syndrome before and three months after decompression. The validity of the PEM questionnaire was compared with the DASH questionnaire and with objective hand function measurements including grip strength, static two-point discrimination and the nine-hole peg test. The responsiveness of the PEM questionnaire following carpal tunnel decompression was also compared with that of the DASH questionnaire. There was a significant correlation between the PEM and DASH questionnaire scores, and between individual questions of the PEM questionnaire and the objective measurements. The PEM questionnaire showed a greater responsiveness to change than the DASH score with an effect size of 0.97 compared with 0.49.

Table 5. Patient Evaluation Measure (PEM) questionnaire

Please put a circle around the number that is the closest to the way you feel about how things have been for you. There are no right or wrong answers.							
Part one- treatment							
1. Throughout my treatment I have seen the same doctor	1	2	3	4	5	6	7
	Every time						Not all the time
2. When the doctor saw me, he or she knew about my case	1	2	3	4	5	6	7
	Very well						Not at all
3. When I was with the doctor, he or she gave me the chance to talk	1	2	3	4	5	6	7
	As much as I wanted						Not at all
4. When I did talk to the doctor, he or she listened and understood me	1	2	3	4	5	6	7
	Very much						Not at all
5. I was given information about my treatment and progress	1	2	3	4	5	6	7
	All that I wanted						Not at all
Part two- how is your hand now? Hand health profile							
1. The feeling in my hand is now	1	2	3	4	5	6	7
	Normal						Absent

Table 5. (Continued)

2. When my hand is cold and/or damp, my hand is now	1	2	3	4	5	6	7
	Non-existent						Unbearable
3. Most of the time, the pain in my hand is now	1	2	3	4	5	6	7
	Non-existent						Unbearable
4. The duration my pain is present is	1	2	3	4	5	6	7
	Never						All the time
5. When I try to use my hand for fiddly things, it is now	1	2	3	4	5	6	7
	Skilful						Clumsy
6. Generally when I move my hand it is	1	2	3	4	5	6	7
	Flexible						Stiff
7. The grip in my hand is now	1	2	3	4	5	6	7
	Strong						Weak
8. For everyday activities, my hand is now	1	2	3	4	5	6	7
	No problem						Useless
9. For my work, my hand is now	1	2	3	4	5	6	7
	No problem						Useless
10. When I look at the appearance of my hand now, I feel	1	2	3	4	5	6	7
	Unconcerned						Embarrassed and self-conscious
11. Generally when I think about my hand I feel	1	2	3	4	5	6	7
	Unconcerned						Very upset
Part three- overall assessment							
1. Generally, my treatment at the hospital has been	1	2	3	4	5	6	7
	Very satisfactory						Very unsatisfactory
2. Generally, my hand is now	1	2	3	4	5	6	7
	Very satisfactory						Very unsatisfactory
3. Bearing in mind my original injury and condition, I feel my hand is now	1	2	3	4	5	6	7
	Better than I expected						Worse than I expected

In 2007, Forward et al studied the validity and internal consistency of the PEM questionnaire in 200 patients with distal radius fracture. They assessed the patients six to forty-two years after injury using the PEM and DASH questionnaires and objective measures of outcome including grip and pinch strength and range of movement. They found highly significant correlations between the PEM and DASH questionnaires, and between the PEM questionnaire and objective measures. One drawback of the study is the use of PEM questionnaires completed for both the injured and uninjured wrist, and then used to calculate a comparative PEM score by subtracting the score of the uninjured wrist from that of the injured side, to eliminate the effect of co-existing disease. This score was found to more strongly correlate with outcome than the PEM score alone. The authors concluded that the PEM questionnaire was a valid method of assessing distal radial fracture outcome.

Michigan Hand Outcome Questionnaire

The Michigan Hand Outcome (MHO) questionnaire assesses hand function, activities of daily living, work performance, pain, aesthetics and satisfaction. The MHO questionnaire, like the DASH, was developed for use in North America. In 1998, Chung et al developed the questionnaire (Table 6) after assessing outcome measures considered important by a panel of patients, hand therapists and hand surgeons. Chung et al describe the development of the questionnaire including the initial psychometric testing, and assessment of the reliability and validity.

The authors used a literature search of pre-existing questionnaires to identify questions related to upper limb function and created a preliminary version of the MHO questionnaire. A panel of patients were also asked to produce relevant questions. This resulted in 100 questions that were then evaluated by a panel of patients, hand therapists and hand surgeons. It was determined that the questions would fall into six domains: overall hand function, activities of daily living, pain, work performance, aesthetics and patient satisfaction with hand function. The preliminary version of the MHO questionnaire was also evaluated by two psychometricians with experience in the designing of questionnaire, and redundant questions were eliminated and wordings modified. Factor analysis was used to further decrease the number of questions in the six domains to 37. Four domains, overall hand function, activities of daily living, aesthetics, and satisfaction with hand function, contain questions for both right and left hand to offset the confounding effect of hand dominance.

After the MHO questionnaire had been revised, it was pilot tested in 200 patients waiting for their first appointment at a hand clinic. The patients also completed a SF-12 questionnaire. To calculate the score, the responses to all questions were added and normalised to a scale from 0 to 100. In the pain domain, a higher score indicates greater pain and a lower score indicates less pain. In the remaining five domains, a higher score indicates better hand function and a lower score indicates poorer hand function. Validity and reliability were tested.

Content or face validity indicates whether the questionnaire appears logical to a group of experts. A panel of patients with hand disorders, hand therapists and hand surgeons evaluated the questionnaire for content validity.

Construct validity assesses the domains in the questionnaire to see if they perform as expected compared with other measures e.g. the SF-12. To investigate the construct validity, the six domains were analysed for correlations with each other. The Spearman's rank correlation showed a high correlation among the five functional domains: overall hand function, activities of daily living, work performance, pain, and satisfaction with hand function. The aesthetics domain however showed a weaker correlation with the other scales with values ranging from -0.29 to 0.46. Only three of the domains in the MHO questionnaire were compared with the SF-12 questionnaire, and these were activities of daily living, work performance and pain. Although the pain domain had a substantial correlation with the pain question in the SF-12, the activities of daily living and work performance domains only had a moderate correlation. To determine the domains that were significant predictors of physical function, all domains were regressed against the physical function component of the SF-12. The activities of daily living, overall hand function and aesthetics domains did not show a significant relation with physical function.

Table 6. Michigan Hand Outcome (MHO) questionnaire.

Instructions: This survey asks for your views about your hands and your health. This information will help keep track of how you feel and how well you are able to do your usual activities. Answer *every* question by marking the answer as indicated. If you are unsure about how to answer a question, please give the best answer you can.					
I. The following questions refer to the function of your hand(s)/wrist(s) *during the past week.* (Please circle I answer for each question.)					
A. The following questions refer to your *right* hand/wrist.					
	Very Good	*Good*	*Fair*	*Poor*	*Very Poor*
1. Overall, how well did your *right* hand work?	1	2	3	4	5
2. How well did your *right* fingers move?	1	2	3	4	5
3. How well did your *right* wrist move?	1	2	3	4	5
4. How was the strength in your *right* hand?	1	2	3	4	5
5. How was the sensation (feeling) in your *right* hand"?	1	2	3	4	5
B. The following questions refer to your *left* hand/wrist.					
	Very Good	*Good*	*Fair*	*Poor*	*Very Poor*
1. Overall, how well did your *left* hand work?	1	2	3	4	5
2. How well did your *left* fingers move?	1	2	3	4	5

Table 6. (Continued)

3. How well did your *left* wrist move?	1	2	3	4	5
4. How was the strength in your *left* hand?	1	2	3	4	5
5. How was the sensation (feeling) in your *left* hand'?	1	2	3	4	5
II. The following questions refer to the ability of your hand(s) to do certain tasks *during the past week.* (Please circle 1 answer for each question.)					
A. How difficult was it for you to perform the following activities using your *right hand?*					
	Not at All Difficult	*A Little Difficult*	*Somewhat Difficult*	*Moderately Difficult*	*Very Difficult*
1. Turn a door knob	1	2	3	4	5
2. Pick up a coin	1	2	3	4	5
3. Hold a glass of water	1	2	3	4	5
4. Turn a key in a lock	1	2	3	4	5
5. Hold a frying pan	1	2	3	4	5
B. How difficult was it for you to perform the following activities using your *left hand?*					
	Not at All Difficult	*A Little Difficult*	*Somewhat Difficult*	*Moderately Difficult*	*Very Difficult*
1. Turn a door knob	1	2	3	4	5
2. Pick up a coin	1	2	3	4	5
3. Hold a glass of water	1	2	3	4	5
4. Turn a key in a lock	1	2	3	4	5
5. Hold a frying pan	1	2	3	4	5
C. How difficult was it for you to perform the following activities using *both of your hands?*					
	Not at All Difficult	*A Little Difficult*	*Somewhat Difficult*	*Moderately Difficult*	*Very Difficult*
1. Open a ,jar	1	2	3	4	5
2. Button a shirt/blouse	1	2	3	4	5
3. Eat with a knife/fork	1	2	3	4	5
4. Carry a grocery bag	1	2	3	4	5
5. Wash dishes	1	2	3	4	5
6. Wash your hair	1	2	3	4	5
7. Tie shoelaces/knots	1	2	3	4	5
III. The following questions refer to how you did in your *normal work* (including both housework and school work) during the past *4 weeks.* (Please circle 1 answer for each question.)					

Table 6. (Continued)

	Always	*Often*	*Sometimes*	*Rarely*	*Never*
1. How often were you unable to do your work because of problems with your hand(s)/wrist(s)?	1	2	3	4	5
2. How often did you have to shorten your work day because of problems with your hand(s)/ wrist(s)?	1	2	3	4	5
3. How often did you have to take it easy at your work because of problems with your hand(s)/wrist(s)?	1	2	3	4	5
4. How often did you accomplish less in your work because of problems with your hand(s)/wrist(s)?	1	2	3	4	5
5. How often did you take longer to do the tasks in your work because of problems with your hand(s)/wrist(s)?	1	2	3	4	5
IV. The following questions refer to how much *pain* you had in your hand(s)/wrist(s) *during the past week* (Please circle 1 answer for each question.)					
1. How often did you have pain in your hand(s)/wrist(s)?	1. Always	2. Often	3. Sometimes	4. Rarely	5. Never
If you answered *never* to *question IV-1* above, please skip the following questions and go to the next section.					
2. Please describe the pain you have in your hand(s)/wrist(s).	1. Very mild	2. Mild	3. Moderate	4. Severe	5. Very severe
	Always	*Often*	*Sometimes*	*Rarely*	*Never*
3. How often did the pain in your hand(s)/wrist(s) interfere with your sleep'?	1	2	3	4	5

Table 6. (Continued)

4. How often did the pain in your hand(s)/wrist(s) interfere with your daily activities (such as eating or bathing)?	1	2	3	4	5
5. How often did the pain in your hand(s)/wrist(s) make you unhappy'?	1	2	3	4	5
V. A. The following questions refer to the appearance (look) of your *right* hand during the past week. (Please circle 1 answer for each question.)					
	Strongly Agree	*Agree*	*Neither Agree Nor Disagree*	*Disagree*	*Strongly Disagree*
1. I was satisfied with the appearance (look) of my *right* hand.	1	2	3	4	5
2. The appearance (look) of my *right* hand sometimes made me uncomfortable in public.	1	2	3	4	5
3. The appearance (look) of my *right* hand made me depressed.	1	2	3	4	5
4. The appearance (look) of my *right* hand interfered with my normal social activities	1	2	3	4	5
B. The following questions refer to the appearance (look) of your *left* hand during the past week. (Please circle 1 answer for each question.)					
	Strongly Agree	*Agree*	*Neither Agree Nor Disagree*	*Disagree*	*Strongly Disagree*
1. I was satisfied with the appearance (look) of my *left* hand.	1	2	3	4	5
2. The appearance (look) of my *left* hand sometimes made me uncomfortable in public.	1	2	3	4	5
3. The appearance (look) of my *left* hand made me depressed.	1	2	3	4	5

Table 6. (Continued)

4. The appearance (look) of my *left* hand interfered with my normal social activities	1	2	3	4	5
VI. A. The following questions refer to your satisfaction with your *right* hand/wrist during the past week. (Please circle 1 answer for each question.)					
	Very Satisfied	*Somewhat Satisfied*	*Neither Satisfied Nor Dis-satisfied*	*Somewhat Dissatisfied*	*Dis-satisfied*
1. Overall function of your *right* hand	1	2	3	4	5
2. Motion of the fingers in your *right* Hand	1	2	3	4	5
3. Motion of your *right* wrist	1	2	3	4	5
4. Strength of your *right* hand	1	2	3	4	5
5. Pain level of your *right* hand	1	2	3	4	5
6. Sensation (feeling) of your *right* Hand	1	2	3	4	5
B. The following questions refer to your satisfaction with your *left* hand/wrist during the past week. (Please circle 1 answer for each question.)					
	Very Satisfied	*Somewhat Satisfied*	*Neither Satisfied Nor Dis-satisfied*	*Somewhat Dissatisfied*	*Dis-satisfied*
1. Overall function of your *left* hand	1	2	3	4	5
2. Motion of the fingers in your *left* Hand	1	2	3	4	5
3. Motion of your *left* wrist	1	2	3	4	5
4. Strength of your *left* hand	1	2	3	4	5
5. Pain level of your *left* hand	1	2	3	4	5
6. Sensation (feeling) of your *left* hand	1	2	3	4	5

Reliability was evaluated using test-retest and internal consistency. For test-retest reliability, patients completed the questionnaire at their first appointment in the clinic and a week later at home. The scores for each domain were correlated for the first and the second time point using interclass correlation. Although they had an overall response rate of 99%, the test-retest reliability was only assessed in 22 patients. Intra-class correlation was used to assess test-retest reliability where a score of 1.0 suggests perfect correlation and a score of 0 suggests no correlation. Test-retest analyses showed excellent correlation for the six domains and all domains except aesthetics had correlation scores over 0.85. The mean difference in the questionnaire scores between the time points was also measured to determine if the scores agreed, and showed excellent agreement suggesting good test-retest reliability. Again, this was only done in 22 patients.

Internal consistency measures the homogeneity of the questions that make up a domain and determine if the questions in the domain are highly correlated with each other. A high inter-item correlation suggests that the questions in a domain are all measuring the same thing. Internal consistency is expressed by Cronbach's alpha that can range from 0 to 1.0, where 1.0 suggests perfect internal consistency and 0 suggests no internal consistency. Generally, Cronbach's alpha values of greater than 0.80 in a domain are considered acceptable and values for the six domains ranged from 0.86-0.97 suggesting excellent internal consistency. The Cronbach's alphas were high in testing for internal consistency. High Cronbach's alphas could also indicate redundancy in the domains, and the authors suggested that efforts to develop a shorter version of the MHO questionnaire should be considered.

Although the authors state that the self-administered questionnaire could be completed in 10 minutes and that patients indicated that it was an acceptable length, our experience differs.

In 2004, Massy-Westropp et al evaluated the validity and reliability of the of the MHO questionnaire for assessing disability in 62 patients with rheumatoid arthritis. Although the MHO provided patient and context-specific information, the Sequential Occupational Dexterity Assessment (SODA) questionnaire provided more impairment information that could readily be compared between patients. The pain domain of the MHO questionnaire correlated well with the Australian Canadian Osteoarthritis Hand Index (AUSCAN) questionnaire (r=0.68). Seventeen patients also repeated the questionnaires within five days showing good reliability. The MHO questionnaire has the advantage that it provides information on both hands, and the authors state that clinicians should decide whether bilateral or unilateral hand function is of interest before choosing a questionnaire. The authors concluded that the MHO questionnaire is valid and reliable for assessment of hand disability in rheumatoid patients.

In 2008, Sambandam et al studied the development, validity, reliability, responsiveness and limitations of six different carpal tunnel syndrome outcome measures including the Boston Carpal Tunnel Questionnaire (BCTQ), MHO questionnaire, DASH questionnaire, PEM questionnaire, clinical rating scale (Historical-Objective (Hi-Ob) scale) and Upper Extremity Functional Scale (UEFS). They concluded that the BCTQ, MHO and PEM questionnaires had good validity, reliability and responsiveness both in the hands of the developers of the questionnaires, as well as independent researchers. They also stated that the DASH questionnaire has a potential role in the assessment of carpal tunnel syndrome but requires more validation in exclusive carpal tunnel patients.

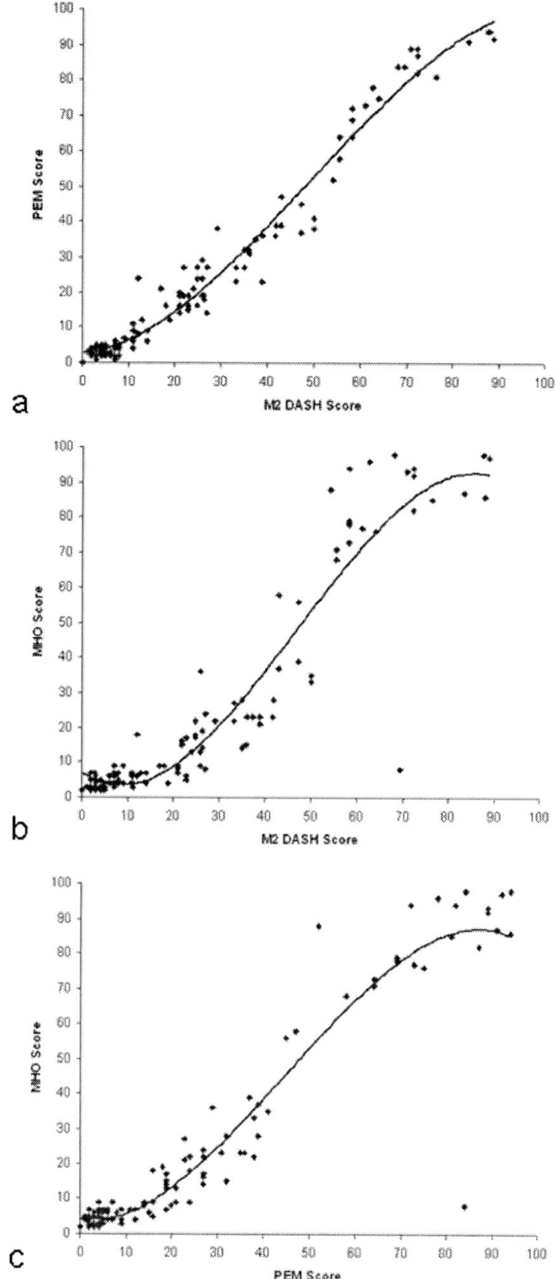

Figure 3. Scatter plots for M2 DASH and PEM scores (a), M2 DASH and MHO scores (b), and PEM and MHO scores (c) (Khan et al, in press).

In 2008, Dias et al studied the construct and criterion validity, reliability, and acceptability of the PEM, MHO and DASH questionnaires in 100 patients with different hand and wrist disorders. They found that the internal consistency of all three questionnaires was very high suggesting some redundancy in questions. They also found that all questionnaires were valid, reliable and reproducible for finger and wrist disorders with a high correlation between the domains. They also studied ease of use using a questionnaire and found that the PEM was the easiest to understand and complete, taking the least time.

The values for the M2DASH, PEM and MHO questionnaires from 40 patients were plot against each other on scatter plots to determine the relationships between them (Khan et al, in press). The M2 DASH and PEM scores showed a fairly linear relationship (Figure 3). The MHO score, when compared to the other two scores, had a more sigmoid shaped curve than linear suggesting that at the extremes, the MHO scores were clustered and not spread out like the M2 DASH and PEM scores. This implies that the MHO score is less sensitive at both extremes.

Conclusion

This chapter does not aim to recommend any one measurement instrument over another, but to provide some basic information regarding questionnaires and an overall assessment of the practicalities and statistical analyses of commonly used region-specific patient-completed questionnaires used in the hand. The choice of instrument to be used will depend on many factors including the project, population and setting, mode of administration, and time and financial constraints. This chapter aims to help researchers identify the advantages and disadvantages of using these questionnaires.

References

[1] Atroshi, I., Gummesson, C., Johnsson, R. & Sprinchorn, A. (1999). Symptoms, disability and quality of life in patients with carpal tunnel syndrome. *J Hand Surg.*, *24*A, 398-404.

[2] Baldry, Currens, J. A. (2000). Evaluation of disability and handicap following injury. *Injury.*, *31*, 99-106.

[3] Beaton, D. E., Katz, J. N., Fossel, A. H., Wright, J. G., Tarasuk, V. & Bombardier, C. (2001). Measuring the whole or the parts? Validity, reliability, and responsiveness of the Disabilities of the Arm, Shoulder and Hand outcome measure in different regions of the upper extremity. *J Hand Ther.*, *14*, 128-146.

[4] Bowling, A. (1997). Research Methods in Health. Open University Press, Buckingham.

[5] Bucher, C., Hume, K. I (2002). Assessment following hand trauma: a review of some commonly employed methods. *Br J Hand Ther.*, *7*, 79-84.

[6] Cano, S. J., Browne, J. P., Lamping, D. L., Roberts, A. H., McGrouther, D. A. & Black N. A. (2004). The Patient Outcomes of Surgery-Hand/Arm (POS-Hand/Arm): a new patient-based outcome measure. *J Hand Surg.*, *29*, 477-485.

[7] Chung, K. C., Pillsbury, M. S. & Walters, M. R. (1998). Reliability and validity testing of the Michigan Hand Outcomes questionnaire. *J Hand Surg.*, *23*A, 575–587.

[8] Cook, D., Guyatt, G., Juniper, E., Griffith, L., McIlroy, W., Willan, A., Jaeschke, R. & Epstein, R. (1993). Interviewer versus self-administered questionnaires in developing health-related quality of life instrument for asthma. *J Clin Epidem.*, *46*, 529-534.

[9] Dias, J. J., Bhowal, B., Wildin, C. J., Thompson, J. R (2001). Assessing the outcome of disorders of the hand. Is the patient evaluation measure reliable, valid, responsive and without bias? *J Bone Joint Surg.*, *83*B, 235-240.

[10] Dias, J. J., Rajan, R. A. & Thompson, J. R. (2008). Which questionnaire is best? The reliability, validity and ease of use of the patient evaluation measure, the disabilities of the arm, shoulder and hand and the Michigan hand outcome measure. *J Hand Surg.*, *33*B, 9-17.

[11] Dowrick, A. S., Gabbe, B. J., Williamson, O. D., Cameron, P. A. (2006). Does the disabilities of the arm, shoulder and hand (DASH) scoring system only measure disability due to injuries to the upper limb? *J Bone Joint Surg.*, *88*B, 524-527.

[12] Drummond, A. S., Sampaio, R. F., Mancini, M. C., Kirkwood, R. N. & Stamm, T. A. (2007). Linking the disabilities of arm, shoulder, and hand to the international classification of functioning, disability, and health. *J Hand Ther.*, *20*, 336-344.

[13] Forward, D. P., Sithole, J. S. & Davis, T. R (2007). The internal consistency and validity of the Patient Evaluation Measure for outcomes assessment in distal radius fractures. *J Hand Surg.*, *32*B, 262-267.

[14] Guyatt, G., Townsend, M., Berman L. & Keller, J. (1987). A comparison of Likert and visual analogue scales for measuring change in function. *J Chron Dis.*, *40,* 1229-1233.

[15] Hervás, M. T., Navarro Collado, M. J., Peiró, S., Rodrigo Pérez, J. L., López Matéu, P. & Martínez Tello, I. (2006). Spanish version of the DASH questionnaire. Cross-cultural adaptation, reliability, validity and responsiveness. *Med Clin* (*Barc*)., *127*, 441-447.

[16] Hobby, J. L., Watts, C. & Elliot, D. (2005). Validity and responsiveness of the patient evaluation measure as an outcome measure for carpal tunnel syndrome. *J Hand Surg.*, *30*B, 350-354.

[17] Imaeda, T., Toh, S., Nakao, Y., Nishida, J., Hirata, H., Ijichi, M., Kohri C. & Nagano A. (2005). for the Impairment Evaluation Committee, Japanese Society for Surgery of the Hand Validation of the Japanese Society for Surgery of the Hand version of the Disability of the Arm, Shoulder, and Hand questionnaire. *J Orthop Sci.*, *10*, 353-359.

[18] Jupiter, J. B. & Ring, D. (2002). Treatment of unreduced elbow dislocations with hinged external fixation. *J Bone Joint Surg.*, *84*A: 1630-1635.

[19] Khan, W. S., Agarwal, M. & Muir, L. (2004). Management of intra-articular fractures of the proximal interphalangeal joint with internal fixation and bone grafting. *Arch Orthop Trauma Surg.*, *124*, 654-658.

[20] Khan, W. S. & Fahmy, N. R. M. (2006). *The S-Quattro in the management of sports injuries of the hand. Injury.*, *37*, 860-868.

[21] Khan, W., Jain, R., Dillon, B., Clarke, L., Fehily, M. & Ravenscroft, M. (2008). The 'M2 DASH'-Manchester-modified Disabilities of Arm Shoulder and Hand score. *Hand*, (N Y). *3*, 240-244.

[22] Khan, W., Dillon, B., Agarwal, M., Fehily, M. & Ravenscroft, M. (2009). The validity, reliability, responsiveness and bias of the Manchester-Modified Disabilities of Arm Shoulder and Hand score in hand injuries. *Hand* (N Y) (in press).

[23] MacDermid, J. C., Richards, R. S., Donner, A., Bellamy, N. & Roth, J. H. (2000). Responsiveness of the short form-36, disability of the arm, shoulder, and hand

questionnaire, patient-rated wrist evaluation, and physical impairment measurements in evaluating recovery after a distal radius fracture. *J Hand Surg.*, *25*A, 330-340.

[24] Macey, A. C., Burke, F. D., Abbott, K., Barton N. J., Bradbury, E., Bradley, A., Bradley, M. J., Brady, O., Burt, A. & Brown, P. (1995).Outcomes of hand surgery. British Society for Surgery of the Hand. *J Hand Surg.*, *20*B, 841-855.

[25] Massy-Westropp, N., Krishnan, J. & Ahern, M. (2004). Comparing the AUSCAN Osteoarthritis Hand Index, Michigan Hand Outcomes Questionnaire, and Sequential Occupational Dexterity Assessment for patients with rheumatoid arthritis. *J Rheumatol.*, *31*, 1996-2001.

[26] McKee, M. D., Wild, L. M. & Schemitsch, E. H. (2003). Midshaft malunion of the clavicle. *J Bone Joint Surg.*, *85*A, 790-797.

[27] Sharma, R. & Dias, J. J. (2000). Validity and reliability of three generic outcome measures for hand disorders. *J Hand Surg.*, *25*B, 593-600.

[28] Streiner, D. & Norman, G. (1994). Health Measurement Scales. Oxford: Oxford University Press.

[29] Westphal, T. (2007). Reliability and responsiveness of the German version of the Disabilities of the Arm, Shoulder and Hand questionnaire (DASH). *Unfallchirurg.*, 110, 548-552.

[30] Wilcke, M. K., Abbaszadegan, H. & Adolphson, P. Y. (2007). Patient-perceived outcome after displaced distal radius fractures: a comparison between radiological parameters, objective physical variables, and the DASH score. *J Hand Ther.*, *20*, 290-299.

[31] Wood-Dauphinee, S. (1999). Assessing quality of life in clinical research: from where have we come and where are we going? *J Clin Epidemiol.*, *52*, 355-363.

In: Hand Surgery: Preoperative Expectations...
Editor: Robert H. Beckingsworth

ISBN: 978-1-60876-280-4

Chapter 3

Principles of Tissue Engineering Approaches for Tendons, Skin, Nerves and Blood Vessels in the Hand

Faizal Rayanmarakkar[1], Wasim S Khan[1*] and Timothy E Hardingham[2]

[1]University College London Institute of Orthopaedics and Musculoskeletal Sciences, Royal National Orthopaedic Hospital, Stanmore, London, HA7 4LP, UK

[2]UK Centre for Tissue Engineering and Wellcome Trust Centre for Cell Matrix Research, Faculty of Life Sciences, University of Manchester, Manchester, M13 9PT, UK

Abstract

Tissue is frequently damaged or lost in injury and disease. There has been an increasing interest in stem cell applications and tissue engineering approaches in surgical practice to deal with damaged or lost tissue. Tissue engineering is an exciting strategy being explored to deal with damaged or lost tissue. It is the science of generating tissue using molecular and cellular techniques, combined with material engineering principles, to replace tissue. This could be in the form of cells with or without matrices. Although there have been developments in almost all surgical disciplines, the greatest advances are being made in orthopaedics, primarily because of familiarity with bone marrow derived mesenchymal stem cells and experience with using materials for scaffolds. Unfortunately significant hurdles remain to be overcome in many areas before tissue engineering becomes more routinely used in clinical practice. In this chapter the tissue engineering

* Corresponding Author: Mr Wasim S Khan, Academic Clinical Fellow, University College London Institute of Orthopaedics and Musculoskeletal Science, Royal National Orthopaedic Hospital, Stanmore, London, HA7 4LP, UK Telephone number: +44 (0) 7791 025554 Fax number: +44 (0) 20 8570 3864 E-mail address: wasimkhan@doctors.org.uk

approaches relevant to hand surgery for tendons, skin, nerves and blood vessels will be discussed.

Introduction

Tissue engineering has been defined as the application of scientific principles to the design, construction, modification and growth of living tissue using biomaterials, cells and factors alone and in combination[33] (Langer and Vacanti, 1993). In essence three elements are central in tissue engineering; stem or precursor cells; an appropriate biological scaffold and growth factors. It generally involves the use of cells with a matrix or scaffold that guides the cells during tissue repair or regeneration. The use of more undifferentiated cell types, such as stem cells or early mesenchymal progenitors that retain multi-lineage and self renewal potential is preferable to the use of terminally differentiated cells. The scaffold could be natural or biosynthetic. Cells harvested from donor tissues, including adult stem cells, can be expanded in culture and associated with resorbable biomaterials forming the scaffold. The cells can be stimulated by specific bioactive molecules such as growth factors. The cells can also be genetically modified via genomic insertion of a new healthy copy of a gene before expansion and subsequent tissue reconstitution. To date the use of gene technology has not been applied to humans. The cells could be stimulated in-vitro to form tissue for future re-implantation in-vivo. Below applications of tissue engineering principles are discussed relevant to tendons, skin, nerves and blood vessels.

1. Tendons

In the united states hand injuries account for 5–10% of annual emergency department visits nationwide and hand surgeons repair nearly one-third of a million digital flexor tendon injuries per year in the United States [48]. Outcome is often unsatisfactory and recovery after surgery takes longer time. Also the repaired tendon regains only half of its initial mechanical properties due to 1) the difficulty to anchorage the tendon in muscle, 2) the high mechanical constraint on the repair structure, 3) the unavailability of ideal tendon grafts, 4) adhesion formation is a major problem, not only in primary repair but also in tendon reconstruction using autografts as well as allografts. Tendon tissue engineering offers an alternative approach to the pitfalls faced in tendon surgery. The main aim is to restore the injured tendon with tissue engineered graft with good structural and functional properties.

Successful repair of ruptured flexor tendons, as measured by restoration of digital flexion function, is a great challenge to hand surgeons because of the lack of adequate donor tendon and flexor tendon adhesions. The first problem arises in loss of tendon substance. The material requirement exceeds availability in devastating injuries although autologous palmaris and plantaris longus tendon grafts are used. The second problem of flexor tendon adhesions is caused by factors like the site and type of injury, the surgical technique and the wound healing response which is most relevant in zone II flexor tendon injuries. The main issue is the 'no-man's land' or Zone II as they are associated with poor prognosis and were treated non-operatively. The biological cascade of events during healing often causes the tendon proper to adhere indiscriminately to its surrounding tissue [37,1]. Clinical and experimental observations suggest that formation of adhesions is precipitated by injury to the tendon sheath, surgical manipulation, and immobilization [18,55,2,3] Extrasynovial tendons are dependent on peripheral neovascularisation, which causes adhesions, but there is a lack of accessible donor intrasynovial tendons for which tissue engineering of intrasynovial tendon grafts would provide a solution to this problem.

The transplantation of a tendon graft is an alternative to primary repair for the hand surgeon. The graft is positioned outside the confines of the flexor sheath in zone II and attached distally in Zone I and proximally in Zone III to the flexor digitorum profundus tendon. Cellular necrosis, inflammation and adhesion may result from routine surgical manipulation of flexor tendon grafts. To address this, devitalised structures such as freeze-dried tendon allografts or tissue-engineered biomaterial scaffolds can be used as alternatives to live autografts in reconstructing the digital flexor mechanism [5].

Tendons are bands of dense connective tissue that help normal joint movement and stability. They protect the muscle (fascia) and fix the length of the muscle belly. They also play a role of damper and shock absorber. They are composed of collagen fibers, and the function and behaviour of tendons depend on of their mechanical properties. They consist of fascicles, fibrils, subfibrils, microfibrils and tropocollagen. Tendon is covered by epitenon which is contiguous paratenon on its outer surface and endotenon on its inner surface. Peritenon with paratenon and epitenon surrounds the tendon and supports gliding. Flexor tendons of the hand are covered by a well defined sheath of synovial cells. Here they (paratenon) are mentioned as tenosynovium, but if there is no synovial lining, the paratenon is called tenovagium. At the musculo-tendinous junction, the perimysium is continuous with the endotenon. At the other extremity on the tendon–bone interface, the collagen fibers and the endotenon become continuous with the periosteum. The tendon insertion into bone is of two types. The first one described by Cooper and Misol shows a transition from the tendon to a layer of fibrocartilage with digitations in the periosteum[16]. Around 50-70% of the tendon is comprised of water and 60-85% of the tendon comprises of type I and type III collagen. Collagen type I is responsible for 70% of the dry weight of the tendon structure. Proteoglycans and leucine-rich protein also play a role in the organisation and mechanical properties of the tissue.

Tendon healing consists of three phases: inflammatory, proliferative and remodeling. During the initial phase of inflammation, fibroblasts and macrophages are recruited to the site of injury, and phagocytosis of the necrotic tissue ensues. During the proliferative phase there is proliferation of fibroblasts and formation of the scar (formed from immature and disorganized collagen matrix). In the final phase of remodelling the immature collagen fibers in the scar tissue become organised and align with the tendon fibers. Therefore the etiology of adhesion formation has been linked to the remodelling phase [37] (Lilly et al 2006).

There are mechanical and biochemical strategies to avoid adhesion formation. Mechanical interventions include post-operative passive motion and rehabilitation protocols post- operatively. Good surgical techniques to minimise the trauma of the tendon, graft, and the surrounding tissues, and the use of anti-adhesion surface coating of the graft as a physical barrier against adhesion formation [40, 8, 25, 41,] (Meislin et al. 1990; Boyer et al. 2005; Hatano et al 2000; Mentzel et al. 2000).

We have to yet define success in creating an ideal tendon substitute using current tissue engineering strategies e.g. synthetic biomaterial scaffolds, in order to improve healing. These engineered scaffolds can be impregnated with genes or growth factors for targeted and timed release at the site of implantation [5] (Basile et al 2008). The main problems are 1) their mechanical strength do not match with those of native tissue, so there is a delay in restoration of function, 2) they do not remodel in response to daily activity, 3) they break down producing by-products that induce inflammation and compromise the repair process [66,5]. Naturally derived materials processed from animal tissue or produced using recombination technology may be better tolerated when implanted [5]. The one that is derived from allogeneic tendon tissue is an ideal example for a naturally derived biomaterial scaffold for tendon tissue engineering. Whitlock et al. had described that a naturally derived biomaterial scaffold from tendon tissue are open to host cell-mediated remodelling and are devoid of cellular material to minimise inflammatory potential. They also possess biomechanical integrity. The tendon designs should allow cell to cell connectivity to allow intracellular communication. Biological and biochemical intervention strategies primarily rely upon growth factor delivery to accelerate the rate of tendon healing and remodelling .While a number of growth factors could potentially improve the repair of tendons, their effects on tendon adhesion have been left largely unexplored [61 19 58 1 29](Towler DA and Gelberman RH 2006; Hsu C and Chang J 2004; Thomopoulos, 2005; Gelberman, 2007; Wang, 2005; Abrahamsson, 1996; Kashiwagi, 2004). A rational design for a growth-factor delivery therapy should be based on the natural history of gene expression of growth factors during the different phases of tendon repair, a thorough understanding of the molecular action of these factors, and a sustained delivery mechanism to maximise the therapeutic effects of these factors.

Tissue engineering techniques have developed biologic and synthetic scaffolds which can repair tendon defects and improve healing by regeneration of the tendon's natural biologic composition to restore its mechanical capacity. One of the most promising scaffold developments from biomechanical and biocompatible points of view would be based on biomimetic strategy. In this approach, the scaffold should include polymeric collagen as the fundamental fibrous phase and being cross linked to give the mechanical strength of the engineered tendon. The combination of scaffold, cell and stimulation, and their applications is the soul of tissue engineering [17] (DeFranco MJ, 2004). This branch also provides new biomaterials that mimic real tissues which induce in vivo regeneration and in vitro functional replacement tissue. The organised collagen structure surrounded by proteoglycans allows tendons to face a wide range of non-linear mechanical deformation which is the main issue in tissue engineering of tendons. Smaller defects are treated by in vivo techniques involving the in situ delivery of genetically modified cells on a scaffold providing immediate mechanical support and boosting the regeneration and healing process. Larger defects or tissue replacement are dealt by in vitro tissue engineering.

Incorporation of cells increases the healing potential of the tendons. Fibroblasts from tendon or skin are used commonly for this purpose. Stem cells are used because of the low mitotic activity of native mature tendon fibroblasts, has proved to be popular. Under mechanical stimulation, MSCs differentiated in fibroblasts, aligned themselves in collagen gel and helped in vivo tendon regeneration. The cells cause gel contraction that improves the biomechanical properties. The cells can be genetically modified to produce growth factors which can amplify healing. DNA synthesis of tendon fibroblasts can be stimulated by treatment with growth factors like PDGF and IGF-1 [4] (Banes et al, 1995). Cross linking (with di-catecholnordihydroguaiaretic acid) and hybridisation (with PLA) techniques have been introduced to augment mechanical properties [31]. Another method is acellular collagen scaffolds, which is in its infancy. Future work in tendon tissue engineering have to focus on biomimetism as defined by Koob (2002) where tendon is engineered by combining scaffold and gene therapy either with cells or with gene activated matrix [31].

2. Skin

Skin, primarily is a protective barrier against the environment and has two layers. The skin is the largest organ of the body comprised of epidermis and dermis with a complex nerve and blood supply. The superficial epidermal layer provides a protection against infection and moisture loss. The deeper dermal layer provides elasticity and mechanical integrity of the skin, and contains the blood vessels that are responsible for the nutrition of the epidermal layer. They constitute the bulk of the skin and are composed of collagen with some elastin and glycosaminoglycans. Major cell type present in the dermis are the fibroblasts and are capable of producing remodelling enzymes such as proteases and collagenases, which play an important role in the wound healing process Appendages like hair follicles or sweat glands, breach the epidermal and dermal layers. Cutaneous sensory nerves pass through the dermal tissue into the epidermal tissue. Regeneration of the epidermis depends on remnants of epidermal cells that lie deep within dermal structures.

When the wound is more than a few cm across, in-growth from the edges of a wound will be insufficient. There is a dire need for skin grafts due to burns, diabetic ulcers and skin cancers. Each year in the United States there are 1.25 million cases of burns, more than 600,000 cases of diabetic ulcers, and another 600,000 cases of skin cancer requiring excision [13, 43] (Brigham, 1996; Mooney, 1999). Majority of them would require skin grafting. Skin grafts were introduced by Reverdin in 1871 and since then various skin substitutes are in vogue. Due to the donor site morbidity associated with autografts and allografts, there is a great deal of demand for an alternative which led to significant advances in tissue engineering of skin e.g. cultured autologous and allogenic keratinocytes grafts, autologous or allogenic composites, acellular biological matrices, and cellular matrices including biological substances such as fibrin sealant. These substitutes ideally should have barrier function, even though none of them have shown better results than autologous split skin grafting. Moreover we have to tide over issues like the need for second procedure, infection, rejection, immune and allergic reaction. At the same time we have to replicate the anatomy, physiology, biologic stability, or aesthetic nature of uninjured skin. The disadvantages of autologous cells are lack of quicker access off-the-shelf for the treatment of burns and trauma. There are three locations from which cell types for skin substitutes can be derived: local, systemic, and progenitor cell populations.

Local cells that could be used for skin tissue engineering applications include fibroblasts, keratinocytes, melanocytes, adipocytes and hair follicle cells. The local quiescent fibroblasts migrate into the affected area, produce extra-cellular matrix proteins, and promote wound contraction. Wound fibroblasts produce extra-cellular matrix proteins including collagen types I and III, fibronectin and proteoglycans, and are responsible for tissue remodelling, scar formation and repair. Systemic cells resident in the blood or bone marrow play a key role in skin wound healing. Progenitor cells are present in hair follicles, bone marrow or could be cultured in vitro from embryonic stem cell line. Keratinocytes can be grown in relatively large numbers over a period of 3 to 4 weeks. They are expensive, are prone to infection and cosmetically poor due to the absence of basement membrane and dermis. Even if their colony forming efficiency is decreased by 50%, cultured epithelial autograft sheets have been stored as frozen suspensions to use them at their optimum. Self-renewing stem cells is a solution to recreate skin and these cells in a keratinocyte culture is all that required for generating epidermal grafts. The significance of dermis in skin healing has led to the development of different engineered skin substitutes e.g. cadaveric skin, collagen based dermal substitute, hyaluronic based membranes, synthetic polymers and composite of biologic and synthetic materials.

Apligraf is a composite derived by combining bovine collagen with fibroblasts with an epidermal layer of neonatal allogeneic keratinocytes. This composite is currently the most sophisticated commercially available tissue-engineered product, and also the most expensive. Its main role is in the treatment of chronic ulcers. Healing is speeded up in chronic wounds [26] (Jones 2002). Clinical applications of acellular human dermal substitute have shown good outcomes in hand and foot burns. It not only retains dermal elements and but also allows migration of keratinocytes [15] (Chong, 2006). Alloderm is processed human cadaveric skin from which the epidermis has been removed and the cellular components of the dermis have been extracted prior to cryopreservation in order to avoid a specific immune response. It is a good template for dermal regeneration. Take rates are good and it reduces scarring of full-thickness wounds and allows grafting of an ultra-thin split-skin graft as a one-stage procedure [26] (Jones 2002). Dermagraft, a cryopreserved living dermal structure, manufactured by cultivating neonatal allogeneic fibroblasts on a polymer scaffold (polyglycolic acid or polyglactin-910, marketed as Dexon or Vicryl, respectively) was developed in order to permanently implant to replace the patient's damaged dermis with a living human material. Dermagraft stimulates the ingrowth of fibrovascular tissue from the wound bed and cause re-epithelialisation from the wound edges.

Clinical failure due to delays in vascularisation is the main drawback of tissue-engineered skin products. Various techniques for increasing vascularisation and promoting wound healing have been developed. One of the methods consists of formation of a matrix comprising gel (denatured collagen) and a nitric oxide inhibitor (L-arginine analog such as N-nitro-L-arginine and D-arginine). The matrix also contains a nitric oxide scavenger, such as dextran, heparin, cysteine, or cystine. A better understanding of the factors influencing extra-cellular matrix formation in tissue-engineering scaffolds is essential to achieve further development in skin generation [70] (Priya et al).

3. Nerve

Nerve regeneration is a complex biological phenomenon and their repair poses a great task as the effects of nerve injury are not localised to the site of injury. Nerves can regenerate on their own if injuries are small in the peripheral nervous system. Surgical treatment is imperative for larger injuries. There is not only functional loss, caused by lack of innervations, but also changes occur along the entire path of the nerve from the target end organ to the central nervous system, with great effect on eventual outcomes [38 42] (Lundborg G. 2000 Merzenich MM, 1983). Advances in neuroscience, cell culture, genetic techniques, and biomaterials have provided optimism for new treatments for nerve injuries. For peripheral nerves, we can use direct end-to end surgical reconnection of the nerve ends or use an autologous graft for a larger nerve defect. Loss of function at the donor site and the need for multiple surgeries are the main drawbacks. There are devices that are now FDA approved for short nerve defects including Integra Neuro sciences Type I collagen tube (NeuraGen Nerve Guide) and SaluMedica's SaluBridge Nerve Cuff [39 3] (Archibald SJ, 1995. Lundborg G, 1997).

Various Treatment Options Are

I. Autologous tissue grafts e.g. nerve grafts, vein grafts, muscle grafts, epineurial sheaths and tendon grafts.
II. Nonautologous/acellular grafts e.g. immunosuppression with allografts, acellular allografts and xenografts, thermal decellularisation, radiation treatment, chemical decellularisation, small intestinal submucosa.
III. Natural-based materials e.g. extra-cellular matrix protein-based material, fibronectin, laminin, collagen and hyaluronic acid-based materials, fibrin/fibrinogen, alginate, agarose.
IV. Synthetic materials. There are various types:

1. Biodegradable synthetic materials e.g. Polylactic acid (PLA), Polylactic-co-glycolic acid (PLGA), Polycaprolactone, Polyurethane, Polyorganophosphazene, Poly 3-hydroxybutyrate, Polyethylene glycol, Biodegradable glass.
2. Electrically active materials e.g. Piezoelectric Electrically conducting material.
3. Nonbiodegradable synthetic materials e.g. Silicone Gore-Tex or ePTFE.

The biologic substitutes e.g. vessels, muscle and tendon are biocompatible and will not induce a notable immune response and provide a support structure to promote cell adhesion and migration. On the downfall there are potential difficulties with isolation and controlled scale-up, they induce changes in the structural properties of the conduit and cause more scar formation and fibrosis [10,20,63] (Walton RL, 1989; Glasby MA, 1986; Brandt J, 1999).

Nonautologous tissue and extracellular matrix (ECM)-based materials has generated a lot of interest. Allogenic and xenogeneic tissues (donor tissue from cadavers and animals respectively) have the advantages that supplies can be large and their use does not require harvest from the patient. However, these tissues possess some risk of disease transmission and must either be used in conjunction with immunosuppressants or must be processed to remove immunogenic components. Many efforts are being made to process intact nonautologous tissue, rendering it less immunogenic for clinical use. These methods focus on removal or destruction of the immunogenic cells and the preservation of the ECM components that are essentially conserved between species. Many different methods have been explored, including thermal techniques, radiation, and chemical processes. Whereas the biodegradable synthetics grafts minimises the risk of late foreign-body response e.g. polyglycolic acid bioabsorbable conduit (Neurotube; Neuroregen LLC, Bel Air, MD) for digital nerve reconstruction showed superior sensory recovery compared with autografts for gaps less than 3 cm [64] (Weber RA, 2000). Schwann cells surround axons and are key players during the process of nerve regeneration. Scaffolds seeded with cultured Schwann cells seem to have improved nerve regeneration processes in experimental models [23,59] (Tohill M, 2004; Guenard V, 1992). The use of cultured Schwann cells has been limited by difficulty in culturing and expanding these cells *in vitro*. Both foetal and adult progenitor neuronal cells have been tried as alternative sources of cells, but these cells also have problems with harvest and expansion. More recently there has been interest in the use of bone-marrow stem cells to populate nerve conduits. At first glance this might seem counterintuitive because Schwann cells are of ectodermal origin and bone-marrow cells are of mesodermal origin, however there is evidence that stem cells can transdifferentiate across other lineages. These cells are promising because they potentially can be harvested in large amounts from bone-marrow aspiration or possibly even venipuncture. Apart from synthetic biodegradable acellular conduits that currently are available for clinical use, other advances in nerve tissue engineering remain experimental. Convincing outcomes data beyond histologic evidence of nerve regeneration needs to be shown in cell-based conduits before they can be translated from bench to bedside. Newer conduits also likely will incorporate elements of the extracellular matrix such as collagen, laminin, and fibronectin which provide cues to guide axonal regeneration and prevent fibrosis [60, 67] (Tong XJ, 1994;Whitworth IH, 1996).

Growth factors such as nerve growth factor, brain-derived neurotrophic factor, acidic and basic fibroblast growth factors, neurotrophin-3, insulin-like growth factor, platelet-derived growth factor, ciliary neurotrophic factor, interleukin-1, and transforming growth factor also may be supplemented to improve the regeneration process [52] (Raivich G, 1993). New advances are likely to come from the field of developmental neurobiology. Unlike adults, in whom neuronal misdirection and incomplete regeneration are features of nerve regeneration, the development process is marked by accurate path-finding of the developing neuron from the central nervous system to its end organs [30] (Koeberle PD, 2004). As knowledge of these guidance cues increases, strategies based on this understanding will enable the development of improved conduits.

4. Blood Vessels

Blood vessels comprise of three layers, from outside to inside the tunica intima, the tunica media and the tunica adventitia. The vascular wall is mainly composed by three types of cells: the endothelial cells that line the tunica intima, the smooth muscle cells that are predominantly located in the tunica media and the adventitial fibroblasts in the tunica adventitia. The integrity of the vessel and mechanical properties are maintained by the endothelial cells and the smooth muscle cells. The endothelial layer not only provides a continuous selective permeable, thrombo-resistant barrier that facilitates laminar blood flow through the blood vessel but also controls vessel tone, platelet activation, adhesion and aggregation, leukocyte adhesion and smooth muscle cell migration and proliferation. Whereas smooth muscle cells play a major role in maintaining elasticity and radial compliance of the vessels by secreting elastic fibres, elastic lamellae and proteoglycans.

The deficiency of graft material due to varicose veins, trauma, prior surgery and the escalating number of reoperations due to the chronic nature of these diseases has led to a high demand of engineered vascular grafts. The incidence of peripheral arterial disease and end-stage renal failure requiring graft is increasing. Also intermediate and long term patency rates in smaller vessels with a calibre of less than 6 mm are poor.

The off-the-shelf availability, harvesting issues, propagation of autologous cells, long cultivation times, the limited conduit length generated in the bioreactors and the need for additional surgical interventions for sourcing autologous cells are the greatest obstacles to the widespread acceptance of tissue engineering technology in clinical practice.

The aim of vascular tissue engineering is to reproduce biocompatible scaffolds. They use autologous cells like endothelial cells, vascular smooth muscle cells (SMCs) and fibroblasts to preclude the complications like thrombogenicity and immunogenicity. Endothelium has antithrombotic, anticoagulant functions and resists intimal hyperplasia. They contribute to construct properties by extracellular matrix production, structural organisation, and contractilability. Genetic manipulation is being tested to improve the proliferation rate of autologous endothelial cells without losing their other properties. Immune rejection is still a major hurdle for allogeneic endothelial and smooth muscle cells. There are two types of stem cells based on their origin, the embryonic and adult stem cells used as cell sources. Embryonic stem cells are still not introduced in clinical application. The main problems are the ethical issues, immunogenic and tumourgenic problems which have to be dealt with before transplantation. Adult stem cells avoid all these issues [70] (Zhang 2007). Fibroblasts too have been used as a cell source in vascular tissue engineering

For the tissue regeneration process the three dimentional structure of scaffold provides an ideal template for cell growth, migration, differentiation, secretion of extracellular matrix proteins and for directing new tissue formation [70] (Zhang 2007). Scaffolds can be either natural proteins, synthetic or biologic polymers. The main aim is to provide vascular cell remodelling and the structural support. Collagen, elastin and fibronectin are the major components of extra-cellular matrix in the body. The first tissue engineered vascular graft by Weinberg and Bell was created using collagen gel. The methods used to strengthen the collagen gel construct are the use of glycation, wrapping the constructs with Dacron mesh or polyurethane film, the use of non-degradable or degradable meshes as sleeves, and the application of dynamic mechanical stimulation.

Synthetic polymers include polyglycolic acid (PGA), poly-L-lactic acid and polyurethanes. Degradation products, degradation time, compliance, .tensile strength, conduit size and configuration can be accurately modified at the point of manufacture to adjust their biocompatibility, degradation rate and elasticity. They are cheap and can be reproduced easily. But synthetic scaffolds do not grow, they lack cell attachment factors and their degradation products may cause intimal hyperplasia. To overcome these setbacks, biologic scaffolds were developed. There are three types of biological scaffold: decellularised allogeneic and xenogeneic blood vessels, decellularised non-vascular conduits and prefabricated extracellular matrices. Decellularisation is achieved chemically by treating with a combination of detergents, enzyme inhibitors and buffers. Decellularisation can be done mechanically by eversion and surface abrasion. They preserve the extra-cellular matrix components like elastin, collagen and glycasminoglycans which are vital for retention of tensile strength, elasticity, endothelial cell adhesion, proliferation, inhibition of smooth muscle cell proliferation (prevents intimal hyperplasia), migration and antithrombotic properties. The main risk of using xenogeneic scaffolds is transmission of animal pathogens [69] (Yow et al, 2006). The mechanical and haemodynamic properties of vascular grafts are crucial for their long-term survival. Bioreactors have been used to produce functional graft in culture with the desired biomechanical properties. Mechanical property of the engineered graft could be controlled by chemical reagents and growth factors e.g. transforming growth factor 1 (TGF-1), insulin, aprotinin, hyaluronan and retinoic acid. Another most exciting option is the rising potential of EPCs which are mobilised into the circulation in response to vessel injury, are significant source of endothelial cells in the face of vascular injury, forming new blood vessels via vasculogenesis [57] (Tepper et al, 2005). They do not have the capacity of self renewal, but they can differentiate into endothelial cells. They can be augmented by statins or erythropoietin to mobilise EPCs to areas of denuded vessels [57] (Tepper et al, 2005).

References

[1] Abrahamsson, SO; Lohmander, S. Differential effects of insulin-like growth factor-I on matrix and DNA synthesis in various regions and types of rabbit tendons. *J Orthop Res,* 1996, 14(3), 370-6.

[2] Andriano, KP; Tabata, Y; Ikada, Y; Heller, J: In vitro and in vivo comparison of bulk and surface hydrolysis in absorbable polymer scaffolds for tissue engineering. *J Biomed Mater Res,* 1999, 48(5), 602-12.

[3] Archibald, SJ; Shefner, J; Krarup, C; Madison, RD. Monkey median nerve repaired by nerve graft or collagen nerve guide tube. *J Neurosci,* 1995, 15(5 Pt 2), 4109-23.

[4] Banes, AJ; Tsuzaki, M; Hu, P; Brigman, B; Brown, T; Almekinders, L; Lawrence, W; T; Fischer, T. PDGF-BB, IGF-I and mechanical load stimulate DNA synthesis in avian tendon fibroblasts in vitro. *J Biomech,* 1995, 28(12), 1505-13.

[5] Basile, P. et al. Freeze-dried tendon allografts as tissue-engineering scaffolds for Gdf5 gene delivery. *Mol Ther,* 2008, 16(3), 466-73.

[6] Bianco, P; Riminucci, M; Gronthos, S; Robey, PG. Bone marrow stromal stem cells: nature, biology, and potential applications. *Stem Cells,* 2001 19(3), 180-92.

[7] Boden, SD. Bioactive factors for bone tissue engineering. *Clin Orthop Relat Res,* (367 Suppl): 1999, S84-94.

[8] Boyer, MI; Goldfarb, CA; Gelberman, RH. Recent progress in flexor tendon healing. The modulation of tendon healing with rehabilitation variables. *J Hand Ther,* 2005, 18(2), 80-5; quiz 86.

[9] Braddock, M; Houston, P; Campbell, C; Ashcroft, P. Born again bone: tissue engineering for bone repair. *News Physiol Sci,* 2001, 16, 208-13.

[10] Brandt, J; Dahlin, LB; Lundborg, G. Autologous tendons used as grafts for bridging peripheral nerve defects. *J Hand Surg [Br],* 1999, 24(3), 284-90.

[11] Breitbart, AS; Grande, DA; Mason, JM; Barcia, M; James, T; Grant, RT. Gene-enhanced tissue engineering: applications for bone healing using cultured periosteal cells transduced retrovirally with the BMP-7 gene. *Ann Plast Surg,* 1999, 42(5), 488-95.

[12] Brekke, JH; Toth, JM. Principles of tissue engineering applied to programmable osteogenesis. *J Biomed Mater Res,* 1998, 43(4), 380-98.

[13] Brigham, PA; McLoughlin, E. Burn incidence and medical care use in the United States: estimates, trends, and data sources. *J Burn Care Rehabil,* 1996, 17(2), 95-107.

[14] Cancedda, R; Bianchi, G; Derubeis, A; Quarto, R. Cell therapy for bone disease: a review of current status. *Stem Cells,* 2003, 21(5), 610-9.

[15] Chong, AK; Chang, J. Tissue engineering for the hand surgeon: a clinical perspective. *J Hand Surg [Am],* 2006, 31(3), 349-58.

[16] Cooper, RR; Misol, S. Tendon and ligament insertion. A light and electron microscopic study. *J Bone Joint Surg Am,* 1970, 52(1), 1-20.

[17] DeFranco, MJ; Derwin, K; Iannotti, JP. New therapies in tendon reconstruction. *J Am Acad Orthop Surg,* 2004, 12(5), 298-304.

[18] Gelberman, RH; Manske, PR. Factors influencing flexor tendon adhesions. *Hand Clin,* 1985, 1(1), 35-42.

[19] Gelberman, RH; Thomopoulos, S; Sakiyama-Elbert, SE; Das, R; Silva, MJ. The early effects of sustained platelet-derived growth factor administration on the functional and structural properties of repaired intrasynovial flexor tendons: an in vivo biomechanic study at 3 weeks in canines. *J Hand Surg [Am],* 2007, 32(3), 373-9.

[20] Glasby, MA; Gschmeissner, SE; Huang, CL; De Souza, BA. Degenerated muscle grafts used for peripheral nerve repair in primates. *J Hand Surg [Br],* 1986, 11(3), 347-51.

[21] Govender, S. et al. Recombinant human bone morphogenetic protein-2 for treatment of open tibial fractures: a prospective, controlled, randomized study of four hundred and fifty patients. *J Bone Joint Surg Am,* 2002, 84-A (12), 2123-34.

[22] Grigolo, B; Roseti, L; Fiorini, M; Fini, M; Giavaresi, G; Aldini, NN; Giardino, R; Facchini, A. Transplantation of chondrocytes seeded on a hyaluronan derivative (hyaff-11) into cartilage defects in rabbits. *Biomaterials,* 2001, 22(17), 2417-24.

[23] Guenard, V; Kleitman, N; Morrissey, TK; Bunge, RP; Aebischer, P. Syngeneic Schwann cells derived from adult nerves seeded in semipermeable guidance channels enhance peripheral nerve regeneration. *J Neurosci,* 1992, 12(9), 3310-20.

[24] Gundle, R; Joyner, CJ; Triffitt, JT. Human bone tissue formation in diffusion chamber culture in vivo by bone-derived cells and marrow stromal fibroblastic cells. *Bone,* 1995, 16(6), 597-601.

[25] Hatano, I; Suga, T; Diao, E; Peimer, CA; Howard, C. Adhesions from flexor tendon surgery: an animal study comparing surgical techniques. *J Hand Surg [Am],* 2000, 25(2), 252-9.

[26] Jones, I; Currie, L; Martin, RA guide to biological skin substitutes. *Br J Plast Surg,* 2002, 55(3), 185-93.

[27] Kadiyala, S; Young, RG; Thiede, MA; Bruder, SP. Culture expanded canine mesenchymal stem cells possess osteochondrogenic potential in vivo and in vitro. *Cell Transplant,* 1997, 6(2), 125-34.

[28] Kale, S; Biermann, S; Edwards, C; Tarnowski, C; Morris, M; Long, MW. Three-dimensional cellular development is essential for ex vivo formation of human bone. *Nat Biotechnol,* 2000, 18(9), 954-8.

[29] Kashiwagi, K; Mochizuki, Y; Yasunaga, Y; Ishida, O; Deie, M; and Ochi, M. Effects of transforming growth factor-beta 1 on the early stages of healing of the Achilles tendon in a rat model. *Scand J Plast Reconstr Surg Hand Surg,* 2004, 38(4), 193-7.

[30] Koeberle, PD., and Bahr, M. Growth and guidance cues for regenerating axons: where have they gone? *J Neurobiol,* 2004, 59(1), 162-80.

[31] Koob, TJ. Biomimetic approaches to tendon repair. *Comp Biochem Physiol A Mol Integr Physiol,* 2002, 133(4), 1171-92.

[32] Kruyt, MC; van Gaalen, SM; Oner, FC; Verbout, AJ; de Bruijn, JD; and Dhert, WJ. Bone tissue engineering and spinal fusion: the potential of hybrid constructs by combining osteoprogenitor cells and scaffolds. *Biomaterials,* 2004, 25(9), 1463-73.

[33] Langer, R; Vacanti, JP. Tissue engineering. *Science,* 1993, 260(5110), 920-6.

[34] Lee, CH; Singla, A; Lee, Y. Biomedical applications of collagen. *Int J Pharm,* 2001, 221(1-2), 1-22.

[35] Lee, KY; Peters, MC; Anderson, KW; Mooney, DJ. Controlled growth factor release from synthetic extracellular matrices. *Nature,* 2000, 408(6815), 998-1000.

[36] LeGeros, RZ. Properties of osteoconductive biomaterials: calcium phosphates. *Clin Orthop Relat Res,* 2002, (395), 81-98.

[37] Lilly, SI; Messer, TM. Complications after treatment of flexor tendon injuries. *J Am Acad Orthop Surg,* 2006, 14(7), 387-96.

[38] Lundborg, GA. 25-year perspective of peripheral nerve surgery: evolving neuroscientific concepts and clinical significance. *J Hand Surg [Am],* 2000, 25(3), 391-414,.

[39] Lundborg, G; Dahlin, L; Dohi, D; Kanje, M; Terada, NA new type of "bioartificial" nerve graft for bridging extended defects in nerves. *J Hand Surg [Br],* 1997, 22(3), 299-303.

[40] Meislin, RJ; Wiseman, DM; Alexander, H; Cunningham, T; Linsky, C; Carlstedt, C; Pitman, M; Casar, RA. biomechanical study of tendon adhesion reduction using a biodegradable barrier in a rabbit model. *J Appl Biomater,* 1990, 1(1), 13-9.

[41] Mentzel, M; Hoss, H; Keppler, P; Ebinger, T; Kinzl, L; Wachter, NJ. The effectiveness of ADCON-T/N, a new anti-adhesion barrier gel, in fresh divisions of the flexor tendons in Zone II. *J Hand Surg [Br],* 2000, 25(6), 590-2.

[42] Merzenich, MM; Kaas, JH; Wall, J; Nelson, RJ; Sur, M; Felleman, D. Topographic reorganization of somatosensory cortical areas 3b and 1 in adult monkeys following restricted deafferentation. *Neuroscience,* 1983, 8(1), 33-55.

[43] Mooney, DJ; Mikos, AG. Growing new organs. *Sci Am,* 1999, 280(4), 60-5.

[44] Muschler, GF; Nitto, H; Matsukura, Y; Boehm, C; Valdevit, A; Kambic, H; Davros, W; Powell, K; and Easley, K. Spine fusion using cell matrix composites enriched in bone marrow-derived cells. *Clin Orthop Relat Res,* 2003, (407), 102-18.

[45] Olmsted, EA; Blum, JS; Rill, D; Yotnda, P; Gugala, Z; Lindsey, RW; Davis, AR. Adenovirus-mediated BMP2 expression in human bone marrow stromal cells. *J Cell Biochem,* 2001, 82(1), 11-21.

[46] Oreffo, RO; and Triffitt, JT. Future potentials for using osteogenic stem cells and biomaterials in orthopedics. *Bone,* 1999, 25(2 Suppl): 5S-9S.

[47] Partridge, KA; Oreffo, RO. Gene delivery in bone tissue engineering: progress and prospects using viral and nonviral strategies. *Tissue Eng,* 2004, 10(1-2), 295-307.

[48] Pennisi, E. Tending tender tendons. *Science,* 2002, 295(5557), 1011.

[49] Perry, CR. Bone repair techniques, bone graft, and bone graft substitutes. *Clin Orthop Relat Res,* 1999, (360), 71-86.

[50] Petite, H; Viateau, V; Bensaid, W; Meunier, A; de Pollak, C; Bourguignon, M; Oudina, K; Sedel, L; Guillemin, G. Tissue-engineered bone regeneration. *Nat Biotechnol,* 2000, 18(9), 959-63.

[51] Quirk, RA; Chan, WC; Davies, MC; Tendler, SJ; Shakesheff, KM. Poly(L-lysine)-GRGDS as a biomimetic surface modifier for poly(lactic acid). *Biomaterials,* 2001, 22(8), 865-72.

[52] Raivich, G; Kreutzberg, GW. Peripheral nerve regeneration: role of growth factors and their receptors. *Int J Dev Neurosci,* 1993, 11(3), 311-24.

[53] Sakkers, RJ; Dalmeyer, RA; de Wijn, JR; van Blitterswijk, CA. Use of bone-bonding hydrogel copolymers in bone: an in vitro and in vivo study of expanding PEO-PBT copolymers in goat femora. *J Biomed Mater Res,* 2000, 49(3), 312-8.

[54] Shin, H; Jo, S; Mikos, AG. Biomimetic materials for tissue engineering. *Biomaterials,* 2003, 24(24), 4353-64.

[55] Silva, MJ; Boyer, MI; Gelberman, RH. Recent progress in flexor tendon healing. *J Orthop Sci,* 2002, 7(4), 508-14.

[56] Stewart, K; Walsh, S; Screen, J; Jefferiss, CM; Chainey, J; Jordan, GR; Beresford, JN. Further characterization of cells expressing STRO-1 in cultures of adult human bone marrow stromal cells. *J Bone Miner Res,* 1999, 14(8), 1345-56.

[57] Tepper, OM; Capla, JM; Galiano, RD; Ceradini, DJ; Callaghan, MJ; Kleinman, ME; and Gurtner, GC. Adult vasculogenesis occurs through in situ recruitment, proliferation, and tubulization of circulating bone marrow-derived cells. *Blood,* 2005, 105(3), 1068-77.

[58] Thomopoulos, S; Harwood, FL; Silva, MJ; Amiel, D; Gelberman, RH. Effect of several growth factors on canine flexor tendon fibroblast proliferation and collagen synthesis in vitro. *J Hand Surg [Am],* 2005, 30(3), 441-7.

[59] Tohill, M; Terenghi, G. Stem-cell plasticity and therapy for injuries of the peripheral nervous system. *Biotechnol Appl Biochem,* 2004, 40(Pt 1), 17-24.

[60] Tong, XJ; Hirai, K; Shimada, H; Mizutani, Y; Izumi, T; Toda, N; and Yu, P. Sciatic nerve regeneration navigated by laminin-fibronectin double coated biodegradable collagen grafts in rats. *Brain Res,* 1994, 663(1), 155-62.

[61] Towler, DA; Gelberman, RH. The alchemy of tendon repair: a primer for the (S)mad scientist. *J Clin Invest,* 2006, 116(4), 863-6.

[62] Urist, MR. Bone: formation by autoinduction. *Science,* 150(698), 893-9, 1965.

[63] Walton, RL; Brown, RE; Matory, WE., Jr; Borah, GL; Dolph, JL. Autogenous vein graft repair of digital nerve defects in the finger: a retrospective clinical study. *Plast Reconstr Surg,* 1989, 84(6), 944-9; discussion 950-2.

[64] Weber, RA; Breidenbach, WC; Brown, RE; Jabaley, ME; Mass, DPA. randomized prospective study of polyglycolic acid conduits for digital nerve reconstruction in humans. *Plast Reconstr Surg,* 2000, 106(5), 1036-45; discussion 1046-8.

[65] Whitaker, MJ; Quirk, RA; Howdle, SM; Shakesheff, KM. Growth factor release from tissue engineering scaffolds. *J Pharm Pharmacol,* 2001, 53(11), 1427-37.

[66] Whitlock, PW; Smith, TL; Poehling, GG; Shilt, JS; Van Dyke, MA. naturally derived, cytocompatible, and architecturally optimized scaffold for tendon and ligament regeneration. *Biomaterials,* 2007, 28(29), 4321-9.

[67] Whitworth, IH; Brown, RA; Dore, CJ; Anand, P; Green, CJ; Terenghi, G. Nerve growth factor enhances nerve regeneration through fibronectin grafts. *J Hand Surg [Br],* 1996, 21(4), 514-22.

[68] Wu, D; Razzano, P; and Grande, D. A. Gene therapy and tissue engineering in repair of the musculoskeletal system. *J Cell Biochem,* 2003, 88(3), 467-81,.

[69] Yow, KH; Ingram, J; Korossis, SA; Ingham, E; Homer-Vanniasinkam, S. Tissue engineering of vascular conduits. *Br J Surg,* 2006, 93(6), 652-61.

[70] Zhang, WJ; Liu, W; Cui, L; Cao, Y. Tissue engineering of blood vessel. *J Cell Mol Med,* 2007, 11(5), 945-57.

In: Hand Surgery: Preoperative Expectations...
Editor: Robert H. Beckingsworth

ISBN: 978-1-60876-280-4

Chapter 4

Principles of Tissue Engineering Approaches for Bone Repair in the Hand

Wasim S Khan*, Faizal Rayanmarakkar and David R Marsh
University College London Institute of Orthopaedics and Musculoskeletal Sciences, Royal National Orthopaedic Hospital, Stanmore, London, HA7 4LP, UK

Abstract

Tissue is frequently damaged or lost in injury and disease. There has been an increasing interest in stem cell applications and tissue engineering approaches in surgical practice to deal with damaged or lost tissue. Tissue engineering is an exciting strategy being explored to deal with damaged or lost tissue. It is the science of generating tissue using molecular and cellular techniques, combined with material engineering principles, to replace tissue. This could be in the form of cells with or without matrices. Although there have been developments in almost all surgical disciplines, the greatest advances are being made in orthopaedics, especially in bone repair. This is due to many factors including the familiarity with bone marrow derived mesenchymal stem cells and bone grafting. Unfortunately significant hurdles remain to be overcome in many areas before tissue engineering becomes more routinely used in clinical practice. In this chapter the tissue engineering approaches relevant to hand surgery for bone repair will be discussed. Significant hurdles however remain to be overcome before tissue engineering becomes more routinely used in surgical practice.

* Corresponding Author: Academic Clinical Fellow, University College London Institute of Orthopaedics and Musculoskeletal Science, Royal National Orthopaedic Hospital, Stanmore, London, HA7 4LP, UK Telephone number: +44 (0) 7791 025554 Fax number: +44 (0) 20 8570 3864 E-mail address: wasimkhan@-doctors.org.uk

Introduction

Regeneration involves replacement of old tissue with new tissue. It occurs readily in the embryo but is slow in most adult tissue. This may be because of the relatively large number of undifferentiated progenitor cells in the embryo (1 in 10,000) compared with adults (1 in 2,000,000) as shown by Haynesworth et al in 1994. Repair mechanisms in post-embryonic tissue, other than bone, result in scar formation instead of tissue regeneration. Repair is more rapid and designed for survival. It involves the inflammatory cell cascade followed by matrix deposition and the remodeling process which attempts to regenerate damaged tissue.

Bone is continually remodeled as a result of the balance between the activities of the osteoclasts and the osteoblasts. Because of the potential of bone to spontaneously regenerate, most bone lesions, such as fractures, heal well with conventional therapy or surgery. The osteogenic process that commences after the inflammatory phase, under the influence of bone-derived bioactive factors, is initiated by precursor cells from the periosteum adjacent to the fracture site. This generates hard callus by intramemembranous bone formation. A bone graft or substitute is often required to assist in orthopaedic surgery healing of a large traumatic or post-surgical defect and of osseous congenital deformities. The majority of bone formation however is by enchondral ossification of the soft callus that appears after infiltrated mesenchymal cells are induced to chondrogenesis. This improved understanding of repair and regeneration has helped with the development of orthopaedic tissue engineering [32] (Kruyt et al, 2004).

Current Treatment

Current surgical treatment of large bone defects falls into two groups; Illizarov method or bone transport and bone graft transplant (auto-, allo-, xeno-grafts, different biomaterial implants). The Illizarov technique entails an osteotomy followed by bone distraction allowing regeneration of bone. The disadvantages include long recovery period and a high complication rate. The clinical gold standard for bone repair is an autologous graft that is effective, but is limited by the availability of sufficient donor tissue and donor site morbidity. As for graft transplants, vascularised autografts are presently mostly used e.g. autografting cancellous bone applying vascularised grafts of the fibula and iliac crest [49] (Perry, 1999). The disadvantages include problems related to anatomical limitations, graft integration, donor site morbidity including infection and haematoma and limitation of size of reconstruction.

Tissue Engineering

Tissue engineering has been defined as the application of scientific principles to the design, construction, modification and growth of living tissue using biomaterials, cells and factors alone and in combination[33] (Langer and Vacanti, 1993). In essence three elements are central in tissue engineering; stem or precursor cells; an appropriate biological scaffold and growth factors. All three are discussed in detail below. It generally involves the use of cells with a matrix or scaffold that guides the cells during tissue repair or regeneration. The use of more undifferentiated cell types, such as stem cells or early mesenchymal progenitors that retain multi-lineage and self renewal potential is preferable to the use of terminally differentiated cells. The scaffold could be natural or biosynthetic. Cells harvested from donor tissues, including adult stem cells, can be expanded in culture and associated with resorbable biomaterials forming the scaffold. The cells can be stimulated by specific bioactive molecules such as growth factors. The cells can also be genetically modified via genomic insertion of a new healthy copy of a gene before expansion and subsequent tissue reconstitution. To date the use of gene technology has not been applied to humans. The cells could be stimulated in-vitro to form tissue for future re-implantation in-vivo.

A tissue engineering approach to treat skeletal defects involves the use of osteoconductive biomaterial scaffolds with osteogenic cell populations and osteoinductive bioactive factors. A possible tissue engineering approach for bone repair is to use autologous bone marrow stem cells (BMSC) loaded on a scaffold [14] (Cancedda et al, 2003). The three constituents are discussed below.

1. Identification of Appropriate Cell Type

Differentiated cells released from adult tissue exhibit a limited proliferation capacity. This has limitations for their expansion in culture and in vitro reconstruction of tissue. Culturing undifferentiated cells (stem cells or progenitor cells) that have a higher proliferative capacity is more promising. Differentiation of these cells can be obtained in vitro by changing the culture conditions after their expansion or by providing a new physiological micro- environment in the transplant area in vivo.

A stem cell is a cell from the embryo, fetus or adult that, under certain conditions, can reproduce for long periods. It can also give rise to specialised cells of body tissues and organs. The use of stem cells from the embryo or fetus has many ethical considerations whereas the use of adult stem cells is generally well accepted by society. An adult stem cell is an undifferentiated or unspecialized cell present in differentiated tissue, which renews itself; and becomes specialized to yield all of the cell types of the tissue from which it was originated. Their progeny includes both new stem cells and committed progenitors with a more restricted differentiation potential. These progenitor cells in turn give rise to more differentiated cell types. The advantages of using stem cells rather than differentiated cells are a higher proliferative capacity, a higher regenerative potential over time and the ability to allow revascularization of the avascular scaffold. Cells with osteoprogenitor features have been isolated from several tissues including periosteum, bone marrow, adipose tissue and retina. The choice of source depends on accessibility, frequency of cells and information of a particular cell system.

Research suggests that stem cells derived from bone marrow (BMSC) can be expanded for a significant number of cell doublings without cell senescence. In vitro multi-differentiation potentials are gradually lost on expansion [14] (Cancedda et al , 2003). The harvest of bone marrow samples is an easy and relatively safe procedure. The bone marrow is a reservoir of multipotent stem cells for mesenchymal tissues. These multipotential stromal stem cells can differentiate into fibroblastic, osteogenic, adipogenic and reticular cells [6] (Bianco et al, 2001). A large number of BMSCs can be obtained in culture. Culture conditions remain essentially the same as the ones originally described by Friedenstein in 1966; however, to increase the yield of osteoprogenitor cells, the effects of several growth factors on proliferation and differentiation of BMSC have been investigated. In addition, human bone marrow osteoprogenitor cells can be isolated and enriched using monoclonal antibodies as selective markers, such as STRO-1 from a CD34+ fraction, SB-10 (reacting with ALCAM), SH-2 (reacting with CD105) and HOP-26 (reacting with CD63) [46 47 56] (Oreffo and Triffitt, 1999; Stewart et al, 1999; Partridge and Oreffo, 2004). FGF-2 supplementation to the culture medium promotes cell proliferation and maintains their multi-lineage potential during expansion [14] (Cancedda et al, 2003).

Intraoperative adult stem cells technologies are being developed to enhance bone repair in delayed or non-union fractures as shown by Muschler et al in 2003 [44]. One in 23,000 adult bone marrow cells is an osteogenic precursor cell. These cells can potentially be separated by selective cell absorption in the operating theatre making viable implants for immediate surgical use. These cells can be combined with a suitable scaffold and used as an alternative to conventional bone autograft. The transplanted osteogenic stem cells can immediately begin to proliferate and lay down new bone matrix without removing the old matrix present in the autograft. The development of these cell based technologies may result in decreased use of conventional bone banks use dead bone to induce new bone formation.

2. Identification of Appropriate Scaffolds

Mesenchymal stem cells alone are unlikely to be sufficient for bone regeneration. Although marrow injections are simple and provide a reduced risk of morbidity, for large skeletal defects, a scaffold of appropriate shape, size and mechanical competence is required for fracture repair. The use of the scaffold or matrix is not only in controlling growth factor and cell delivery but also to provide a structural template to fill the tissue lesion. These could be naturally occurring or synthetic polymers or bioceramics. Biodegradable scaffolds provide t e initial structure and stability for tissue formation but degrade as tissue forms, providing room for matrix deposition and tissue growth. They can be used alone or in combination with growth factors or osteoconductive materials.

The scaffold aims to mimic the extracellular matrix in a regenerating bone enviromnent. It has to be informative to the cells as well as provide mechanical support. A biomaterial should easily integrate with the adjacent bone and favour new tissue ingrowth (osteo-conduction). It should allow colonization by the host blood vessels, be biocompatible and resorbable.

Polymers include collagen that can be prepared in solution or shaped into membrane films, threads, sponges and acidic hydrogels. It is derived from xenogenic sources and purification techniques are used to eliminate the immunogenic telopeptides. The primary obstacle to their use is the possibility of xenozoonoses [34] (Lee et al, 2001). Heparin-coating fibrin hydrogels can be used to slowly and regularly deliver growth factors with heparin binding affinity such as FGF-2. Alginates extracted from brown algae form a brown lattice hydrogel. It has large average mesh size allowing easy diffusion of macromolecules. Hyaluronic acid binds specifically to proteins. Its stability is increased by partial esterification making it particularly suitable for peptide release or protein delivery [22] (Grigolo et al, 2001).

Synthetic polymers include poly lactic acid (PLA), polyglycolic acid (PGA) and their co-polymer polylactic-co-glycolic acid (PLGA). They allow a better control of physicocliemical properties and delivery kinetics. They also reduce the risk of potential biohazardous complications. The disadvantages are the induction of some immune or inflammatory response after implantation. These polymers are currently used for a number of orthopaedic devices including suture anchors and interference screws) Other biodegradable materials for bone tissue engineering include Degrapol-foam and Polyactive that support bone cell adhesion and proliferation [53] (Sakkers et al, 2000). Surface eroding polymers, such as polyortho-esters may have advantages in load bearing bone applications as only the surface of these materials degrades leaving the bulk the mechanical strength [2] (Andriano et al, 1999).

Bioceramics act as a pre-existing bone surface on which bone cells deposit new bone matrix. Best results so far have been with porous bioceramics and BMSC. Bioceramics made from hydroxyapatite and tricalcium phosp ate are used for bone repair. They have osteoconductive properties and ability to integrate with bone tissue. They are not themselves osteoinductive and are resorbed relatively slow. Their resorbability can be increased by increasing the concentration of tricalcium phosphate. The production of porous scaffolds makes the interna architecture similar to that of cancellous bone. Advantages include large surface available for tissue regeneration and cell delivery and a favorable micro-environmental effect due to the presence of a mineralized matrix [36] (LeGeros, 2002). Problems include biodegradability and inflammatory and immunological reactions [46] (Oreffo and Triffitt, 1999).

Alternative scaffolds are derived from cadavers or animal skeletons and natural scaffolds for example the coral cytoskeleton. Mesenchymal stem cells mixed with coral implants have been shown to stimulate bone regeneration and achieve bone regeneration and achieve bone clinical union in an animal model of bone defect [50 (Petite et al, 2000). Biomimetic material chemistry attempts to reproduce the complex structures that occur in nature, such as coral, nacre and calcite shells and sea urchin spines, in synthetic systems and generate accurate and specific biomaterials. They potentially mimic many roles of the extracellular matrix by providing biological cues for cell-matrix interactions promoting tissue growth. They are modified with bioactive molecules and can be used as tissue engineering scaffolds that potentially serve as an artificial extracellular matrix providing biological cues to guide new tissue formation. More information on immunoreactivity and biocompatibility will be needed before clinical evaluation [54] (Shin et al, 2003).

Smart materials, for example, Arg-Gly-Asp (RGD) sequence peptides involved in integrin mediated cell adhesion can be incorporated onto the scaffold surface to enhance cell adhesion and spreading [51] (Quirk et al, 2001). Drug delivery techniques such as entrapment within a hydrogel matrix allowing growth factor to be released in a controlled fashion from the scaffold to aid the regenerating tissue have been applied [65] (Whitaker et al, 2001). This strategy has been applied in bone tissue engineering where growth factors such as recombinant human bone morphogenetic protein-2, basic fibroblast growth factor and vascular endothelial growth factor have all been successfully incorporated into a hydrogel prior to in vivo implantation [35] (Lee et al, 2000). A future goal will be the introduction of calcium based scaffolds that can gradually degrade at the same rate at which new bone is formed.

3. Growth Factors and Gene Therapy

Growth factors are cytokines that are secreted by many cell types and function as signaling molecules. Members of the TGF beta family, notably bone morphogenetic proteins (BMPs), are particularly relevant to skeletal tissue engineering. Other agents known to induce bone formation include FGF, PDGF and IGF-1, Indian sonic hedgehog and parathyroid hormone. One function of BMP is to induce the differentiation of undifferentiated mesenchymal cells into chondrogenic and osteogenic cells and to promote their proliferation (Saito and Takaota, 2003). BMPs have a role in bone development and thus their incorporation into tissue engineered scaffolds and delivery systems [7] (Boden, 1999).

The isolation of growth factors such as TGF beta 3 and its analogues such as BMPs e.g. BMP 2 and 7 has led to their use to enhance and accelerate bone repair and to replace the bone. Bone induction to assist and enhance bone deposition and repair was first introduced by Marshall Urist in 1965, and led to the isolation of BMPs, which could stimulate osteogenic precursor mesenchymal stem cells (MSCs) to form bone [62]. Human cDNA BMP 7 was cloned in 1990 and recombinant human form followed. It was shown to induce bone formation in animals by stimulating precursor MSCs. Recombinant human BMPs (rhBMPs) have been commercially available for over a decade but their bioavailability, bioactivity and costs have limited their clinical uptake. There are three methods by which BMPs can be used in bone tissue engineering and these include (a) cell therapy (b) gene therapy (c) cytokine therapy (Saito and Takaota, 2003).

Earlier examples include the use of porous PLGA scaffolds with high molecular weight hyaluronic acid for rhBMP-2 delivery [12] (Brekke and Toth, 1998). hnplantation of such constructs into long bone defects promoted cortical bone formation in vivo in rabbits (Mori et al, 2000). Another approach is to use collagens, the favoured carrier for BMPs, to generate composites with hydroxyapatite or PLA for use with rhBMP-2 for tissue engineering. This has shown to be successful in vivo by Winn et al in 1999: TGF beta 1 has been shown to stimulate the three-dimentional cellular development of human bone ex vivo [28] (Kale et al, 2000).

In 2002, injecting the rhBMP-7 into a bone non-union site resulted in healing of the site after 30 months as shown by Giltaij et al. The protein acts by recruiting adult osteogenic precursor MSCs. In a study by Giltaij et al 163 patients with non-union 23 months after injury received the recombinant protein implant and achieved clinical union in 70% andradiological union in 65% by 19 months. No significant adverse reactions were attributed to the implant. There was also a decreased incidence of osteomyelitis at the surgical site and decreased use of post-operative analgesia. A prospective randomized controlled trial of 450 patients concluded that the clinical use of rhBMP-2 as an adjunct to standard management of long bone fractures was safe, well tolerated and showed earlier functional recovery [21]] (Govender et al, 2002).

Gene therapy is the science of the transfer of genetic material into individuals for therapeutic purposes by altering cellular function or structure at the molecular level. The ability to transfer genes into multipotent mesenchymal stem cells has many applications. Developments in gene technology offer the possibility of genetic modification of isolated and expanded cells to produce populations of progenitor cells over-expressing selected signaling molecules. The various techniques and methods currently available to enable gene transfer into a target population include viral methods (transduction) and nonviral methods (transfection). Viral delivery systems used for bone engineering include the retroviral and adenoviral systems. The advantages of viral expression of genes are a high efficiency of transduction (50-100%). The disadvantages include the potential for mutagenesis, carcinogenesis and the immune response to viral infection or proteins. Nonviral gene delivery makes use of lipopolyfection reagents such as liposomes, cationic lipids or cationic polymers complexed with a foreign DNA for transfection. Alternatively they can use physical methods such as microinjection, gene gun delivery or the use of uncomplexed plasmid DNA. The nonviral methods are safer but less efficient and some can cause immunological reactions [47] (Partridge and Oreffo, 2004). Another approach is to use matrices for gene or protein delivery. These provide a stable and sustained release include allogenic cortical bone and synthetic substances [9] (Braddok et al, 2001; Saito and Takaota, 2003).

Gene delivery can be direct in vivo or indirect ex vivo. The direct method involves transferring the genetic material into the target somatic cell in vivo. This is technically simpler to perform in a clinical setting. The indirect technique involves removal of cells from the patient, genetic modifications of the cells ex vivo and return of the cells to the patient. This is technically more complex but is relatively safer and allows for selection of cells for gene expression [68] (Wu et al, 2003). Lieberman et al have shown regional cell and gene therapy using BMP-2 producing bone marrow cells on the repair of segmental bone defects in rats. Brietbant et al have cultured periosteal cells retrovirally transduced with BMP-7 in a polyglycolic acid (PGA) scaffold in a critical sized calvarial defect model in rabbits [11]. Olmsted et al have indicated the potential to generate human bone marrow stromal cells expressing BMP-2 by adenoviral infection [45].

Bone Repair

The aim has been to provide the reconstructed segment with appropriate initial mechanical properties while encouraging new bone formation in the region. Bone formation by BMSC transplanted into small animals was first demonstrated by Friedenstein in 1966. Implanting BMSC combined with 3D mineralized bioceramic scaffolds subcutaneously into immunodeficient mice can be used to assess bone formation. Autologous BMSC and bioceramic composites have been used to repair experimentally induced bone defects (full thickness gaps in tibial diaphysis) in sheep. Gross morphology, radiographs and histology show complete integration of ceramic with bone and good functional recovery. Culture expanded bone marrow cells can heal a segmental bone defect following reimplantation

(Kadiyala et al, 1997) and can give rise to osteogenic tissue within diffusion chambers in a variety of animal species (Gundle et al, 1995) [24, 27]. Similar results with carol scaffold and hydroxyapatite and beta tri-calcium phosphate scaffold have been described. The osteoprogenitor cells were harvested from the iliac crest and expanded in culture.

Based on the above pre-clinical trials, in 2001, autologous osteoprogenitor cells isolated from the bone marrow of patients and expanded in vitro were delivered in vivo with a microporous hydroxyapatite scaffold. This was for patients with 4-7 cm bone detects for whom a traditional therapeutic alternative was difficult or had previously failed. External fixation was provided initially for stability. By the second month, abundant callus formation along the implant and good integration at the interface with the bone were observed. No major complication was observed. All patients recovered limb function in 6-12 months. In cases where bone defects occur in positions requiring dynamic strength, such as long bones of the legs, an alternative to using an external fixator is BMP and polymer composites combined with solid materials with good affinity for bone. For instance a titanium implant with a porous surface on which the BMP and polymer composites are placed. This can be implanted into the bone defect and bone will form on the composite (Saito and Takaota, 2003).

References

[1] Abrahamsson, SO; Lohmander, S. Differential effects of insulin-like growth factor-I on matrix and DNA synthesis in various regions and types of rabbit tendons. *J Orthop* Res, 1996, 14(3), 370-6.

[2] Andriano, KP; Tabata, Y; Ikada, Y; Heller, J. In vitro and in vivo comparison of bulk and surface hydrolysis in absorbable polymer scaffolds for tissue engineering. *J Biomed Mater Res,* 1999, 48(5), 602-12.

[3] Archibald, SJ; Shefner, J; Krarup, C; Madison, RD. Monkey median nerve repaired by nerve graft or collagen nerve guide tube. *J Neurosci,* 1995, 15(5 Pt 2), 4109-23.

[4] Banes, AJ; Tsuzaki, M; Hu, P; Brigman, B; Brown, T; Almekinders, L; Lawrence, W. T; Fischer, T. PDGF-BB, IGF-I and mechanical load stimulate DNA synthesis in avian tendon fibroblasts in vitro. *J Biomech,* 1995, 28(12), 1505-13.

[5] Basile, P. et al. Freeze-dried tendon allografts as tissue-engineering scaffolds for Gdf5 gene delivery. *Mol Ther,* 2008, 16(3), 466-73.

[6] Bianco, P; Riminucci, M; Gronthos, S; Robey, PG. Bone marrow stromal stem cells: nature, biology, and potential applications. *Stem Cells,* 2001, 19(3), 180-92.

[7] Boden, SD. Bioactive factors for bone tissue engineering. *Clin Orthop Relat Res,* 1999, (367 Suppl), S84-94.

[8] Boyer, MI; Goldfarb, CA; Gelberman, RH. Recent progress in flexor tendon healing. The modulation of tendon healing with rehabilitation variables. *J Hand Ther,* 2005, 18(2), 80-5; quiz 86.

[9] Braddock, M; Houston, P; Campbell, C; Ashcroft, P. Born again bone: tissue engineering for bone repair. *News Physiol Sci,* 2001, 16, 208-13.

[10] Brandt, J; Dahlin, LB; Lundborg, G. Autologous tendons used as grafts for bridging peripheral nerve defects. *J Hand Surg [Br],* 1999, 24(3), 284-90.

[11] Breitbart, AS; Grande, DA; Mason, JM; Barcia, M; James, T; Grant, RT. Gene-enhanced tissue engineering: applications for bone healing using cultured periosteal cells transduced retrovirally with the BMP-7 gene. *Ann Plast Surg,* 1999, 42(5), 488-95,.

[12] Brekke, JH; Toth, JM. Principles of tissue engineering applied to programmable osteogenesis. *J Biomed Mater Res,* 1998, 43(4), 380-98.

[13] Brigham, PA; McLoughlin, E. Burn incidence and medical care use in the United States: estimates, trends, and data sources. *J Burn Care Rehabil,* 1996, 17(2), 95-107.

[14] Cancedda, R; Bianchi, G; Derubeis, A; Quarto, R. Cell therapy for bone disease: a review of current status. *Stem Cells,* 2003, 21(5), 610-9.

[15] Chong, AK; Chang, J. Tissue engineering for the hand surgeon: a clinical perspective. *J Hand Surg [Am],* 2006, 31(3), 349-58.

[16] Cooper, RR; Misol, S. Tendon and ligament insertion. A light and electron microscopic study. *J Bone Joint Surg Am,* 1970, 52(1), 1-20.

[17] DeFranco, MJ; Derwin, K; Iannotti, JP. New therapies in tendon reconstruction. *J Am Acad Orthop Surg,* 2004, 12(5), 298-304.

[18] Gelberman, RH; Manske, PR. Factors influencing flexor tendon adhesions. *Hand Clin,* 1985, 1(1), 35-42.

[19] Gelberman, RH; Thomopoulos, S; Sakiyama-Elbert, SE; Das, R; Silva, MJ. The early effects of sustained platelet-derived growth factor administration on the functional and structural properties of repaired intrasynovial flexor tendons: an in vivo biomechanic study at 3 weeks in canines. *J Hand Surg [Am],* 2007, 32(3), 373-9.

[20] Glasby, MA; Gschmeissner, SE; Huang, CL; De Souza, BA. Degenerated muscle grafts used for peripheral nerve repair in primates. *J Hand Surg [Br],* 1986, 11(3), 347-51.

[21] Govender, S. et al. Recombinant human bone morphogenetic protein-2 for treatment of open tibial fractures: a prospective, controlled, randomized study of four hundred and fifty patients. *J Bone Joint Surg Am,* 2002, 84-A(12), 2123-34.

[22] Grigolo, B; Roseti, L; Fiorini, M; Fini, M; Giavaresi, G; Aldini, N. N; Giardino, R; and Facchini, A. Transplantation of chondrocytes seeded on a hyaluronan derivative (hyaff-11) into cartilage defects in rabbits. *Biomaterials,* 2001, 22(17), 2417-24.

[23] Guenard, V; Kleitman, N; Morrissey, TK; Bunge, RP; Aebischer, P. Syngeneic Schwann cells derived from adult nerves seeded in semipermeable guidance channels enhance peripheral nerve regeneration. *J Neurosci,* 1992, 12(9), 3310-20.

[24] Gundle, R; Joyner, CJ; Triffitt, JT. Human bone tissue formation in diffusion chamber culture in vivo by bone-derived cells and marrow stromal fibroblastic cells. *Bone,* 1995, 16(6), 597-601.

[25] Hatano, I; Suga, T; Diao, E; Peimer, CA; Howard, C. Adhesions from flexor tendon surgery: an animal study comparing surgical techniques. *J Hand Surg [Am],* 2000, 25(2), 252-9.

[26] Jones, I; Currie, L; Martin, R. A guide to biological skin substitutes. *Br J Plast Surg,* 2002, 55(3), 185-93.

[27] Kadiyala, S; Young, RG; Thiede, MA; Bruder, SP. Culture expanded canine mesenchymal stem cells possess osteochondrogenic potential in vivo and in vitro. *Cell Transplant,* 1997, 6(2), 125-34.

[28] Kale, S; Biermann, S; Edwards, C; Tarnowski, C; Morris, M; and Long, MW. Three-dimensional cellular development is essential for ex vivo formation of human bone. *Nat Biotechnol,* 2000, 18(9), 954-8.

[29] Kashiwagi, K; Mochizuki, Y; Yasunaga, Y; Ishida, O; Deie, M; Ochi, M. Effects of transforming growth factor-beta 1 on the early stages of healing of the Achilles tendon in a rat model. *Scand J Plast Reconstr Surg Hand Surg,* 2004, 38(4), 193-7.

[30] Koeberle, PD; Bahr, M. Growth and guidance cues for regenerating axons: where have they gone? *J Neurobiol,* 2004, 59(1), 162-80.

[31] Koob, TJ. Biomimetic approaches to tendon repair. *Comp Biochem Physiol A Mol Integr Physiol,* 2002, 133(4), 1171-92.

[32] Kruyt, MC; van Gaalen, SM; Oner, FC; Verbout, AJ; de Bruijn, JD; Dhert, WJ. Bone tissue engineering and spinal fusion: the potential of hybrid constructs by combining osteoprogenitor cells and scaffolds. *Biomaterials,* 2004, 25(9), 1463-73.

[33] Langer, R; Vacanti, JP. Tissue engineering. *Science,* 1993, 260(5110), 920-6.

[34] Lee, CH; Singla, A; and Lee, Y. Biomedical applications of collagen. *Int J Pharm,* 2001, 221(1-2), 1-22.

[35] Lee, KY; Peters, MC; Anderson, KW. Mooney, DJ. Controlled growth factor release from synthetic extracellular matrices. *Nature,* 2000, 408(6815), 998-1000.

[36] LeGeros, RZ. Properties of osteoconductive biomaterials: calcium phosphates. *Clin Orthop Relat Res,* 2002, (395), 81-98.

[37] Lilly, SI; Messer, TM. Complications after treatment of flexor tendon injuries. *J Am Acad Orthop Surg,* 2006, 14(7), 387-96.

[38] Lundborg, G. A 25-year perspective of peripheral nerve surgery: evolving neuroscientific concepts and clinical significance. *J Hand Surg [Am],* 2000, 25(3), 391-414,.

[39] Lundborg, G; Dahlin, L; Dohi, D; Kanje, M; Terada, N. A new type of "bioartificial" nerve graft for bridging extended defects in nerves. *J Hand Surg [Br],* 1997, 22(3), 299-303.

[40] Meislin, RJ; Wiseman, DM; Alexander, H; Cunningham, T; Linsky, C; Carlstedt, C; Pitman, M; Casar, R. A biomechanical study of tendon adhesion reduction using a biodegradable barrier in a rabbit model. *J Appl Biomater,* 1990, 1(1), 13-9.

[41] Mentzel, M; Hoss, H; Keppler, P; Ebinger, T; Kinzl, L; Wachter, NJ. The effectiveness of ADCON-T/N, a new anti-adhesion barrier gel, in fresh divisions of the flexor tendons in Zone II. *J Hand Surg [Br],* 2000, 25(6), 590-2.

[42] Merzenich, MM; Kaas, JH; Wall, J; Nelson, RJ; Sur, M; Felleman, D. Topographic reorganization of somatosensory cortical areas 3b and 1 in adult monkeys following restricted deafferentation. *Neuroscience,* 1983, 8(1), 33-55.

[43] Mooney, DJ; Mikos, AG. Growing new organs. *Sci Am,* 1999, 280(4), 60-5.

[44] Muschler, GF; Nitto, H; Matsukura, Y; Boehm, C; Valdevit, A; Kambic, H; Davros, W; Powell, K; Easley, K. Spine fusion using cell matrix composites enriched in bone marrow-derived cells. *Clin Orthop Relat Res,* 2003, (407), 102-18.

[45] Olmsted, EA; Blum, JS; Rill, D; Yotnda, P; Gugala, Z; Lindsey, RW; Davis, AR. Adenovirus-mediated BMP2 expression in human bone marrow stromal cells. *J Cell Biochem,* 2001, 82(1), 11-21.

[46] Oreffo, RO; Triffitt, JT. Future potentials for using osteogenic stem cells and biomaterials in orthopedics. *Bone,* 1999, 25(2 Suppl), 5S-9S.

[47] Partridge, KA; Oreffo, RO. Gene delivery in bone tissue engineering: progress and prospects using viral and nonviral strategies. *Tissue Eng,* 2004, 10(1-2), 295-307.

[48] Pennisi, E. Tending tender tendons. *Science,* 2002, 295(5557), 1011.

[49] Perry, CR. Bone repair techniques, bone graft, and bone graft substitutes. *Clin Orthop Relat Res,* 1999, (360), 71-86.

[50] Petite, H; Viateau, V; Bensaid, W; Meunier, A; de Pollak, C; Bourguignon, M; Oudina, K; Sedel, L; and Guillemin, G. Tissue-engineered bone regeneration. *Nat Biotechnol,* 2000, 18(9), 959-63.

[51] Quirk, RA; Chan, WC; Davies, MC; Tendler, SJ; Shakesheff, KM. Poly(L-lysine)-GRGDS as a biomimetic surface modifier for poly(lactic acid). *Biomaterials,* 2001, 22(8), 865-72.

[52] Raivich, G; Kreutzberg, GW. Peripheral nerve regeneration: role of growth factors and their receptors. *Int J Dev Neurosci,* 1993, 11(3), 311-24.

[53] Sakkers, RJ; Dalmeyer, RA; de Wijn, JR; van Blitterswijk, CA. Use of bone-bonding hydrogel copolymers in bone: an in vitro and in vivo study of expanding PEO-PBT copolymers in goat femora. *J Biomed Mater Res,* 2000, 49(3), 312-8.

[54] Shin, H; Jo, S; Mikos, AG. Biomimetic materials for tissue engineering. *Biomaterials,* 2003, 24(24), 4353-64.

[55] Silva, MJ; Boyer, MI; Gelberman, RH. Recent progress in flexor tendon healing. *J Orthop Sci,* 2002, 7(4), 508-14.

[56] Stewart, K; Walsh, S; Screen, J; Jefferiss, CM; Chainey, J; Jordan, GR; Beresford, JN. Further characterization of cells expressing STRO-1 in cultures of adult human bone marrow stromal cells. *J Bone Miner Res,* 1999, 14(8), 1345-56.

[57] Tepper, OM; Capla, JM; Galiano, RD; Ceradini, DJ; Callaghan, MJ; Kleinman, ME; and Gurtner, GC. Adult vasculogenesis occurs through in situ recruitment, proliferation, and tubulization of circulating bone marrow-derived cells. *Blood,* 2005, 105(3), 1068-77.

[58] Thomopoulos, S; Harwood, FL; Silva, MJ; Amiel, D; Gelberman, RH. Effect of several growth factors on canine flexor tendon fibroblast proliferation and collagen synthesis in vitro. *J Hand Surg [Am],* 2005, 30(3), 441-7.

[59] Tohill, M; Terenghi, G. Stem-cell plasticity and therapy for injuries of the peripheral nervous system. *Biotechnol Appl Biochem,* 2004, 40(Pt 1), 17-24,.

[60] Tong, XJ; Hirai, K; Shimada, H; Mizutani, Y; Izumi, T; Toda, N; Yu, P. Sciatic nerve regeneration navigated by laminin-fibronectin double coated biodegradable collagen grafts in rats. *Brain Res,* 1994, 663(1), 155-62.

[61] Towler, DA; Gelberman, RH. The alchemy of tendon repair, a primer for the (S)mad scientist. *J Clin Invest,* 2006, 116(4), 863-6.

[62] Urist, MR. Bone: formation by autoinduction. *Science,* 150(698), 893-9, 1965.

[63] Walton, RL; Brown, RE; Matory, WE., Jr; Borah, GL; Dolph, JL. Autogenous vein graft repair of digital nerve defects in the finger: a retrospective clinical study. *Plast Reconstr Surg,* 1989, 84(6), 944-9; discussion 950-2.

[64] Weber, RA; Breidenbach, WC; Brown, RE; Jabaley, ME; Mass, DP. A randomized prospective study of polyglycolic acid conduits for digital nerve reconstruction in humans. *Plast Reconstr Surg,* 2000, 106(5), 1036-45; discussion 1046-8.

[65] Whitaker, MJ; Quirk, RA; Howdle, SM; Shakesheff, KM. Growth factor release from tissue engineering scaffolds. *J Pharm Pharmacol,* 2001, 53(11), 1427-37.

[66] Whitlock, PW; Smith, TL; Poehling, GG; Shilt, JS; Van Dyke, M. A naturally derived, cytocompatible, and architecturally optimized scaffold for tendon and ligament regeneration. *Biomaterials,* 2007, 28(29), 4321-9.

[67] Whitworth, IH; Brown, RA; Dore, CJ; Anand, P; Green, CJ; Terenghi, G. Nerve growth factor enhances nerve regeneration through fibronectin grafts. *J Hand Surg [Br],* 1996, 21(4), 514-22.

[68] Wu, D; Razzano, P; Grande, DA. Gene therapy and tissue engineering in repair of the musculoskeletal system. *J Cell Biochem,* 2003, 88(3), 467-81.

[69] Yow, KH; Ingram, J; Korossis, SA; Ingham, E; Homer-Vanniasinkam, S. Tissue engineering of vascular conduits. *Br J Surg,* 2006, 93(6), 652-61.

[70] Zhang, WJ; Liu, W; Cui, L; Cao, Y. Tissue engineering of blood vessel. *J Cell Mol Med,* 2007, 11(5), 945-57.

In: Hand Surgery: Preoperative Expectations...
Editor: Robert H. Beckingsworth

ISBN: 978-1-60876-280-4

Chapter 5

Motion Preserving Procedures for Degenerative Osteoarthritis of the Wrist due to Advanced Carpal Collapse

L. De Smet[*] and I. Degreef
[1]Department of Orthopedic Surgery U.Z. Pellenberg
Weligerveld, 1 B-3212 Lubbeek (Pellenberg) Belgium

Abstract

Arthrodesis of the wrist has been considered as the gold standard for osteoarthritis of the wrist. In 1984 Watson and Ballet [1] recognized a specific pattern of carpal collaps (SNAC), other alternatives have been proposed: the proximal row carpectomy (PRC) and the scaphoidectomy combined with a four corner arthrodesis. In this cohort of 54 patients, two motion preserving procedures were compared (26 PRC's and 28 four corner fusions)

The PRC had significantly better outcome for range of motion and DASH. Grippping force was not significantly different between both procedures

Keywords: wrist, arthrodesis, SLAC/SNAC, proximal row carpectomy

Introduction

A lot has been written on the degenerative osteoarthritis of the wrist due to advanced carpal collapse since the pattern has been described in 1984 by Watson & Ballet [1].

[*] Correspondence author: Department of Orthopedic Surgery, U.Z. Pellenberg, Weligerveld, 1, B-3212, Lubbeek (Pellenberg), Belgium, Tel.: 016/338800, Fax: 016/338803, E-mail. luc.desmet@uz.kuleuven.ac.be

Several operative treatment options have been evocated: complete or partial arthrodesis, resection or prosthetic arthroplasty and denervation All have been reported as valuable procedures. None of the comparative series between proximal row carpectomy (PRC) and the four corner procedure could demonstrate a significant difference [2-9]. Vanhove et al in 2008 [8] confirmed this, but found a shorter perion of work incapacity for PRC compared to the four corner arthrodesis

The purpose of this paper is to compare the clinical outcome for four corner arthrodesis (4CA) and for PRC.

Material and Methods

Patients

We reviewed all patients who were treated for degenerative osteoarthritis of the wrist due to advanced carpal collapse: scapholunate advanced collapse (SLAC) and scaphoid non-union advanced collapse (SNAC). Fifthy four patients with 54 involved wrist could be retrieved: 26 with a PRC and 28 with a 4CA. There were 43 men and 11 women with a mean age of 52 years (range 28 to 74 y). The right side was involved 32 times, the left 22 times. There were 17 SNAC wrists and 37 SLAC wrists. There were no significant differences concerning age, gender distribution, pathology and involved sides between the patients into the two groups (Table 1). Minimum follow up was 12 months (range 12 – 72).

The PRC group consisted of 26 patients, 4 women, 22 males with a mean age of 48 years (SD 13.6), 14 right wrists, 12 left wrists; 9 for a SNAC (scaphoid nonunion advanced collaps and 17 for a SLAC (scapholunate advanced collaps) wrist, all stage 2. Seventeen wore at work (15 blue collars, 2 white collars

28 patients, 7 women, 21 men with 4CA were evaluated. The mean age was 55,2 years (range 28-74).. Twenty right wrists and 8 left wrists were involved; 20 SLAC and 8 SNAC-wrists; 13 patients were at work (9 blue collars and 4 white collars).

The choice of procedure was mainly determinated by the surgeons preference. PRC was judged not indicated when severe damage on the head of the capitate was radiologically visible; minor cartilaginous damage on the capitate observed during the a PRC did not change the planned interventention. The surgical procedures have been described previously by several authors.

Surgical Technique

PRC. Surgery was performed under either regional or general anesthesia. A dorsal longitudinal incisions incorporating existing scars was used. The extensor retinaculum was identified and divided over the third compartment. The EPL was mobilized radialy, the fourth compartiment with the EDC tendons was mobilsed without opening it ulnarly. The wrist capsule was identified and a ligament sparing capsulotomy according to Berger et al [10] was performed. The proximal row was inspected. If no significant degenerative changes were present, the PRC procedure was performed. Sharp division of the intercarpal ligaments facilitated mobilization of the bones. The lunate was first removed, followed by the scaphoid and triquetrum. The palmar capsule and extrinsic radiocarpal ligaments were preserved. Passive flexion and extension of the hand were done in neutral and slight radial deviation to detect impingement of the trapezium against the radial styloid. Five patients required a radial styloidectomy. The capsule and extensor retinaculum were closed anatomically. Temporary pinning of the radiocarpal joint, soft-tissue interpositional arthroplasty or resection of the proximal pole of the capitate was not performed. Post-operative immobilization with cast or splint varied from 0 to 8 weeks. Thumb and finger motion were started immediately. After removing the casts, active wrist motion was started. Physiotherapy was only applied if there was a significant rigidity after 6 weeks.

4CA: The wrist was approached dorsally and the ligament sparing capsulotomy is used to explore the carpus [10]. The scaphoid was freed from adherences and removed. The articular cartilage between the lunate, capitate, triquetrum and hamate bones was removed. A K-wire in the dorsal lunate was used as a joystick to correct the dorsal intercalated segmaent instability (DISI) and temporary fixed. In twenty six cases we used the resected scaphoid as autologous bone graft. In two cases autologous crista iliaca spongious bone graft were used. Four methods of fixation were used: Herbert® screws (11 cases) (Zimmer, Warsaw, IN, USA), K-wire (5 cases), staples (once) and Spider® plate (KMI, San Diego, CA, USA). (11 times) The wrist was immobilized for 6 weeks in a below elbow cast.

Evaluation

The follow-up examination was performed by independent observers not involved in the patients treatments: they asked for patients satisfaction (more than 75% satisfied with the procedure or not?). Physical examination included flexion, extension, ulnar deviation and radial deviation measured with a hand holded goniometer on both wrists and compared with preoperative values. Grip force was measured with Jamar® Dynamometer

For evaluation of the disability, the DASH-score [11](disability of the arm, shoulder and hand, Dutch language version [12]) and the PRWE (patient rating wrist evaluation) [13] for evaluating the outcome. The PRWE function score consists of 10 questions scores from 0 to 10 and the overall result is calculated and scored from 0 to 100. The PRWE pain score consists of the five questions (scored from 0 to 50).

Table 1. Summary data of the cohort.

	N	Mean age	Range age	M/F	SLAC/SNAC	Side L/R
PRC	26	48	28-71	22/4	17/9	12/14
4 CA	28	55	28-74	21/7	20/8	8/20

Table 2. a) outcome (DASH) and range of motion (ROM) (mean SD)

	Satisfaction	DASH	Extension/flexion
PRC	16/10	16 (16.8)	44° (14.7) / 37° (14.7)
4 CA	8/11	39 (30.9)	52° (12) / 32° (13)

Table 2b. Gripping force: mean (standard deviation)

	Preop force	Postop force	contralateral
PRC	22 (11.7)	31 (26.8)	42 (11.0)
4CA	24 (5.7)	24 (12.0)	36 (16.3)

(PRC = proximal row carpectomy, 4CA = four corner arthrodesis, RCA = radiocarpal arthrodesis)

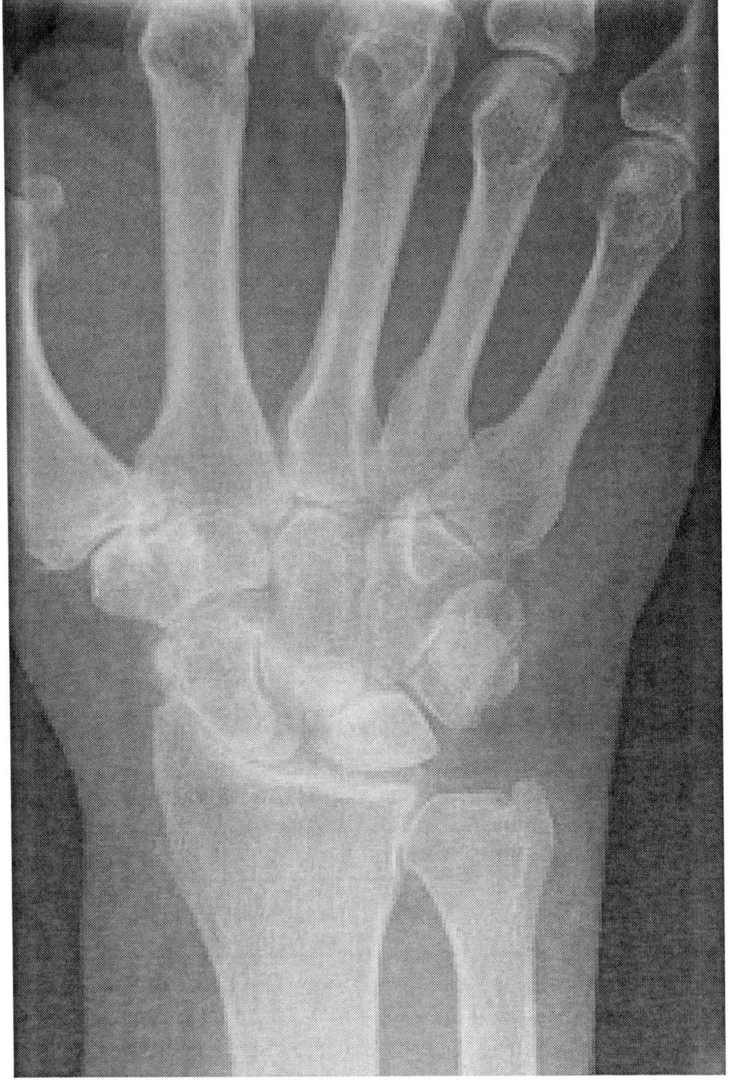

Figure 1. (Continued)

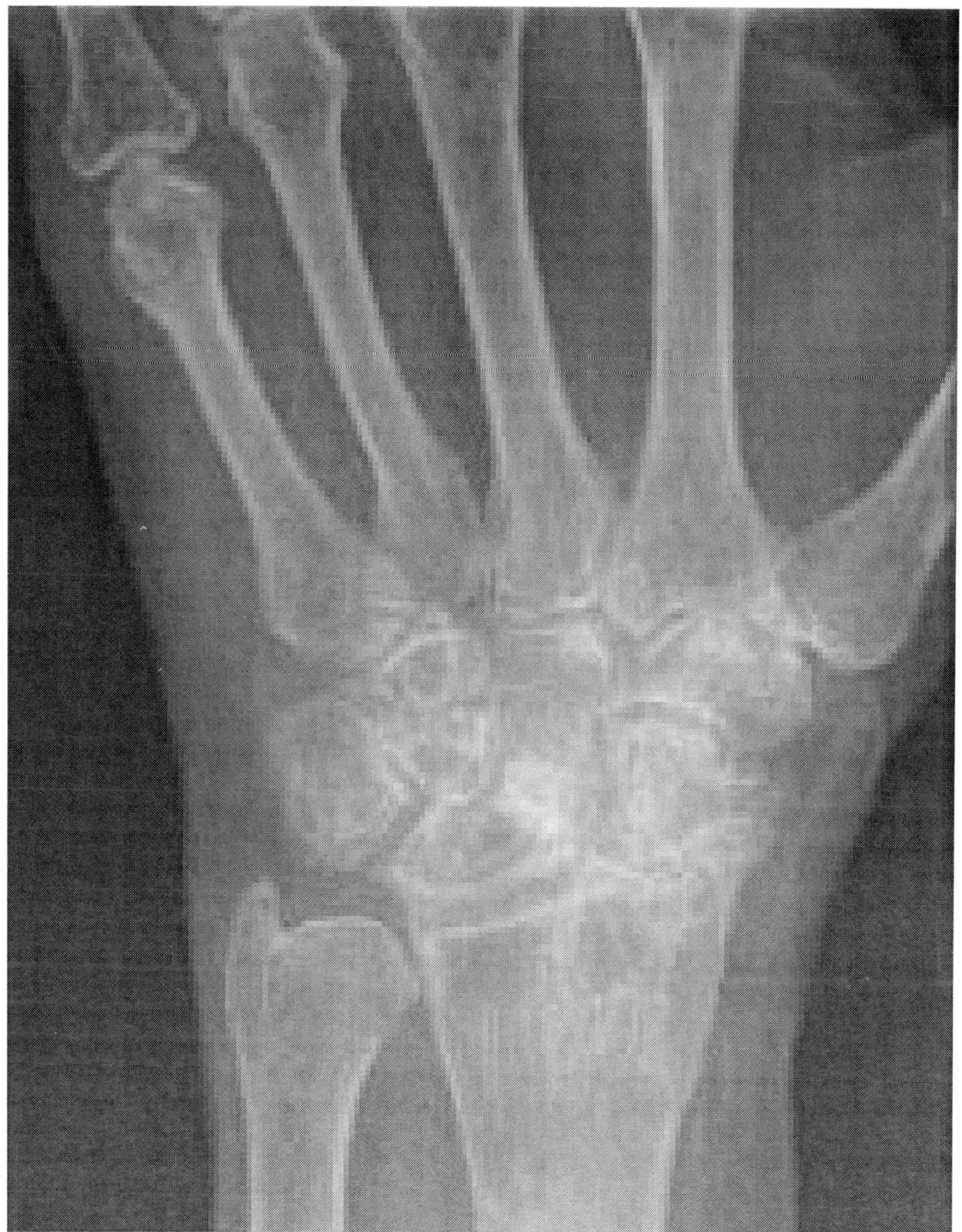

Figure 1. SLAC wrist (scapholunate advanced collpas) with good preservation of the joint between lunate and radius. (a) Stage 2 with preserved capitolunate joint. (b) stage 3 with destroyed capitolunate joint

All data were analyzed and compared with chi square test and students't-test and paired T-test. Significancy was set at $p < 0.05$.

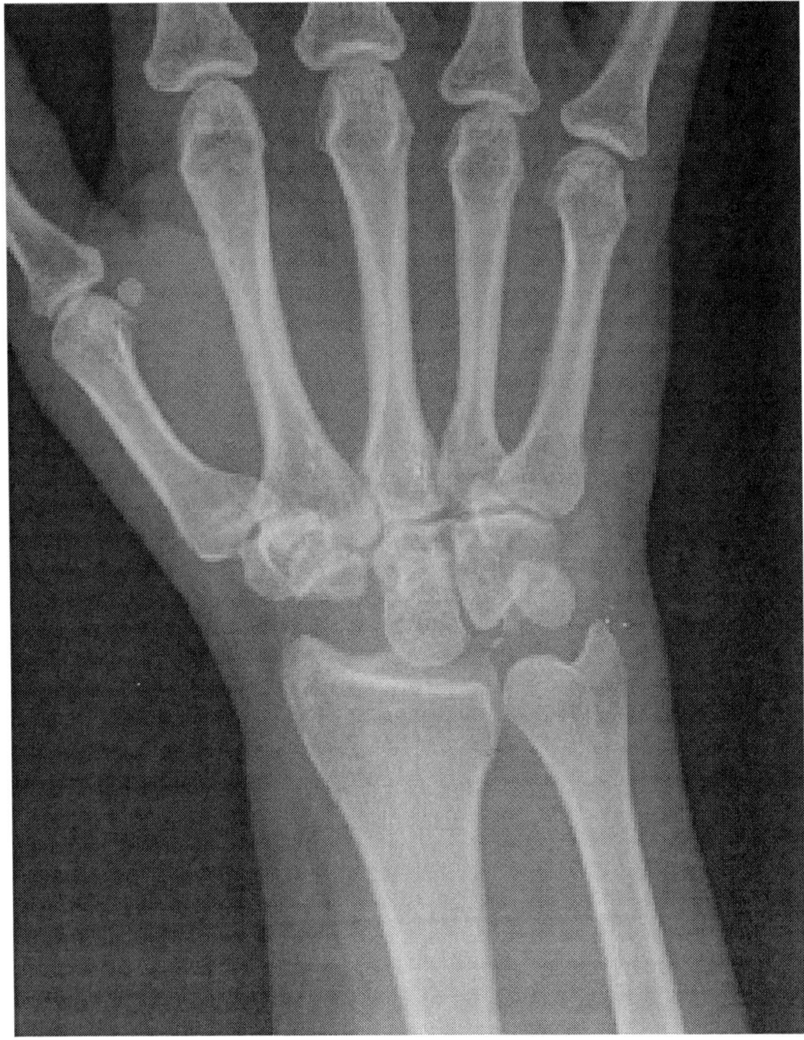

Figure 2. Status after proximal row carpectomy

Results

The Results Are Summarized In Tables 2

In the PRC group 18 were fully satisfied, 8 were not. The range of motion in PRC is considerable: 64° extension (SD 11.5) and 37° flexion (SD 13.0). The gripping force, 31 kg (SD 26.8) still remains weaker than the contralateral side: on average 74%. The increase in gripping force was significant ($p = 0.025$), from 22 kg (SD 11,7) (52%) to 31kg (SD 26.8) (74%). The DASH score was 16 (SD 16.8). PRWE was 23/100 (SD 23.1) Complications were few and minor, none no secondary operations were necessary. Patients could regain their job at 27 weeks (SD 14.4, range 11 to 56 weeks, one was on permanent compensation) after PRC. White collar workers regained their work after 14 weeks, blue collar workers after 29 weeks.

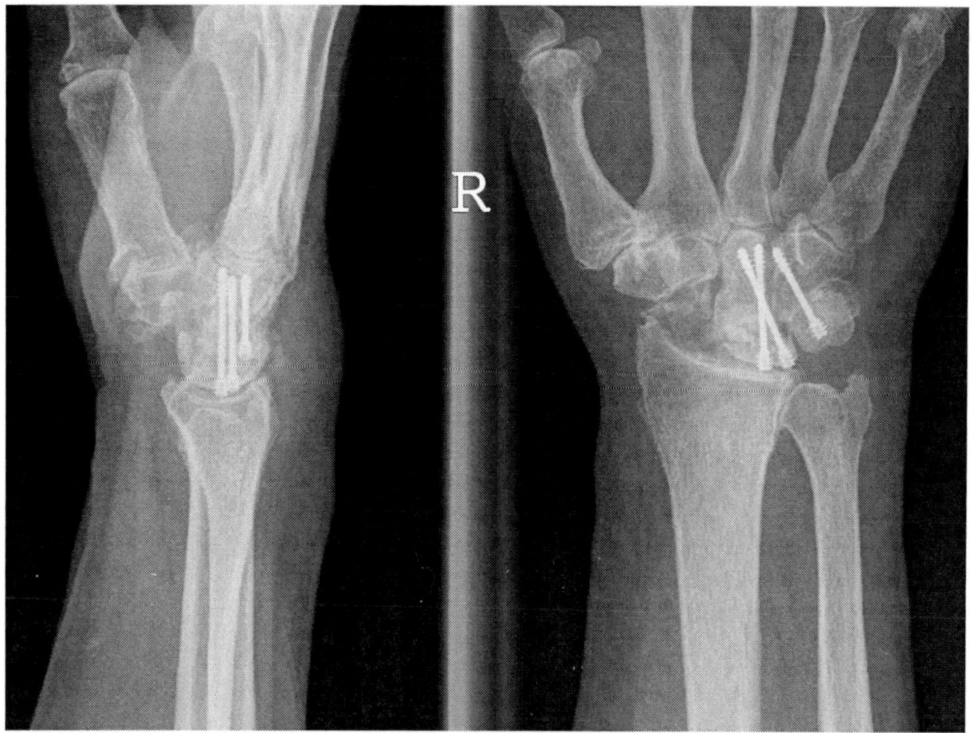

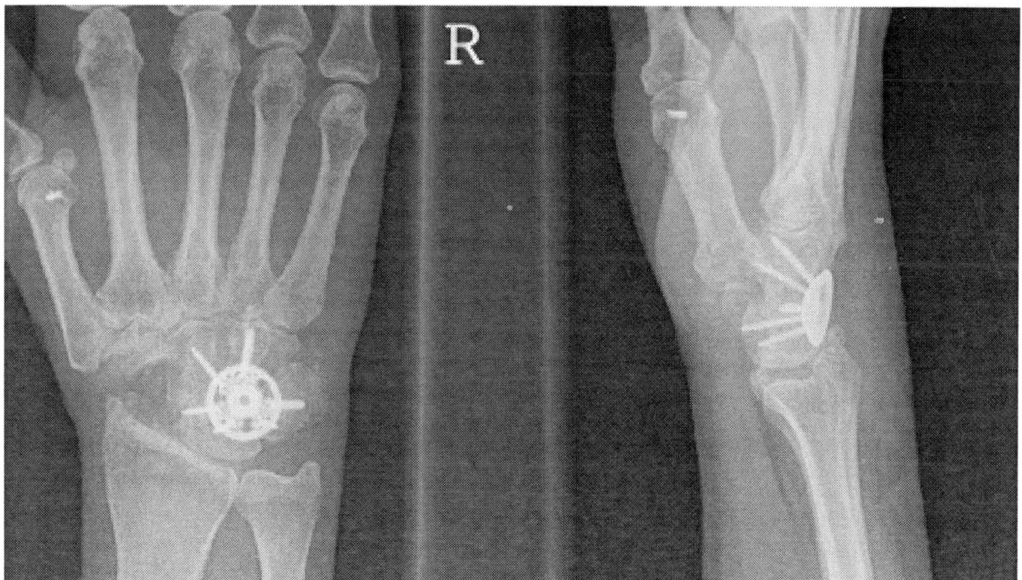

Figure 3. Status after 4 corner arthrodesis

Nineteen patients with a 4CA had no pain during everyday activities, 4 patients had moderate pain and 5 patients had frequent pain during daily activities, none had pain at rest. In the 4CA, xx were satisfied, xx0 were not.. The mean preoperative range of flexion was 36° (range 5° - 60°) (SD 13,8); at follow up it was 29° (range 10° - 60°) (SD 12,5). This difference is significant (p = 0.052) (t-test). The mean preoperative range of extension was

36° (range 5° - 65°) (SD 16,3); at follow-up it was 23° (range 0° - 58°) (SD 11.9) ($p < 0.01$) (paired T-test). Mean preoperative grip strength increased from 47% to 72% postoperatively (not significant $p = 0.13$). The mean absolute value postoperatively was 24 kg (SD 11.9). The postoperative DASH score was 39 (range 2 – 98) (SD 30,9)(Table 1). Postoperative PRWE function score was 40/100 (range 0 – 96, SD 27.8). There were 3 complications: one pin tract infection, one perforation of a screw, one neuropraxia of the radial nerve. The mean duration of working incapacity was 23 weeks (SD 17.1, range 4 to 56 weeks, 2 were on permanent compensation) Of the 9 blue collar workers: 1 was on permanent compensation, 5 regained their original job, 3 had to switch to a lighter manual job. Their mean duration of work incapacity was 29 weeks. The white collar workers were off work for 11 weeks

The DASH scores were significantly differrent in favour for the PRC (T-test, $p<0.001$) There was a significant correlation between the DASH score and the gripping force at follow-up: ($p=0.046$ with a correlation coefficient $r = -0.39$). However the gripping forces were not significantly different between the 2 groups ($p = 0.2$) Probably due to the large variation (and thereby the high standard deviation). The PRWE was significantly better in PRC compared to 4CA (t-test, $p = 0.018$)

The ranges of motion after PRC and 4CA were into the functional ranges. Between these 2 groups the values were significantly different ($p < 0.001$ for extension, $p = 0.036$ for flexion) (t-test) in favour of the PRC. Only in the PRC group there was a significant increase between preoperative and postoperative values ($p<0.006$, paired T test).

Discussion

During decades and still now in numerous publications and textbooks, total wrist (radiocarpometacarpa)l arthrodesis was considered as the gold standard for unresolved wrist problems. For most insurance companies this statement is favorable since this is the "administrative" end of a sometimes long history.

The outcome of wrist arthrodesis has been studied by several authors. Their results have varied widely and the outcome probably depends on socio-economic provisions, the composition of the patient cohort and the outcome assessment used by the author(s) [14-25]. However there have been more critical voices [26-29] drawing the attention to the poor patient satisfaction and the long periods of working incapacity

The question of how much motion is needed is not fully answered. It is not clear to which extent some motion of the wrist is useful or necessary. In most impairment tables there is a linear relationship between motion and impairment. Some authors have measured the range of motion (ROM) during activities of daily life (ADL). The values were highly variable. Palmer et al [30] claimed that 5° of flexion and 30° of extension were functional ROM's, Brumfield and Champoux [31] claimed 10° of flexion and 15° of extension while the measurements of Ryu et al [32] found a much higher ROM, 60° of extension and 54° flexion. Nelson [33] approached the problem from another viewpoint: the measured to required motion to perform the ADL with or without problems, 11° of ROM resulted in a slight disability in 13 of the 125 ADL's. Adams et al [34] reproduced these simulated wrist restriction in volunteers and concluded that perceived disability was higher than measured functional loss with conventional physical tests.

In a personal study survey we concentrated on the disability rather than the impairment. In a large group of operated patients with several procedures the impact of reduced ROM (and gripping force) was correlated to the disability. There was only a weak correlation with DASH and ROM indicating that preservation of some ROM was more important than the amount of ROM. [35]

PRC converts a complex link joint system to a simple hinge joint by creating a radio-capitate articulation. The result is not physiologic and normal kinetics should not be expected, but clinical results are satisfactory in most follow-up series [36-63]. Jebson et al [48] revealed only a trend toward an increasing prevalence and degree of osteoarthritis with longer follow-up evaluation: range of postoperative motion reported in prior studies has been variable, ranging from 40% to 60% of the unaffected side. Radial deviation was consistently been the most reduced. A major criticism of PRC is weakness that is believed to be secondary to the mechanical effect of the relative tendon lengthening. A large literature review has been reported by Nagelvoort et al in 2002 [52]. They found the mean gripping force varying between 60 and 100 % of the opposite side. Trackle et al in 2003, obtained only 54% gripping force [61]. In our series it was 70% [40] Only the recent articles mention the DASH score; it ranges between 9 and 36. [5,41,52,59,61]. A large series in our own department of 50 patients with a minimum follow-up of one year found a DASH score of 18 [40]

In 1984 Watson and Ballet [1] described the SLAC pattern and proposed the scaphoid replacement by a silicone spacer combined with a 4CA. Lateron, due to the ongoiing problems with silicone implants, scaphoid excision was proposed rather than replacement. Since then numerous investigators have reported favorable outcome of this procedure [64-71].

A few authors compared a PRC with a partial arthrodesis (scaphoidectomy and 4-corner arthrodesis), none of them observed significant differences [2-9]. Tomaino et al in 1994 [7] compared 15 patients with a PRC with 9 patients with a limited wrist fusion. Range of motion was significantly better after PRC; pain relief and gripping forca were only minimally different. In the same year Krakauer et al [3] found a similar result: better range of motion in PRC, gripping force was better in 4CA, but statistical signoficancy was not mentioned. Similar findings in the paper of Wyrick et al [9], all outcome measures (pain relief, range of motion an d gripping force) in favor of the PRC but none of them significant. Cohen and Kozin [2] found only minimal differences between the group of 19 patients with a PRC compared to the 19 patients with a 4CA Krimmer et al in 2000 [4] compared RCA with 4CA and found no significant difference in DASH score (33 for 4CA in 97 patients and 45 in RCA for 41 patients) and both groups were satisfied (respectively 86 and 84%). Vanhove et al [8] compared 15 patients with a PRC and 15 with a 4CA. No differences were found except for the duration of hodpitamstay and working incapacity all in favor for the PRC. Lukas et al [5] found a beter DASH score for the 4CA (12 patients), but range of motion, force and pain relief were similar with the PRC (14 patients). For kienbock's disease, Nakamura et al [6] concluded that limited wrist fusions (13 cases) gave a better outcome than PRC (20 cases), but this pathology is completely different from the SLAC/SNAC.

The good outcome of published series of PRC could be confirmed. The loss of gripping power after PRC and the restoration of gripping power after arthrodesis has not been confirmed.

This is the first survey which demonstrates that PRC is better than partial arthrodesis, although prospective randomized investigations however are required for confirmation. The weakness of this study is its retrospective character and the possible bias in indication, but is is the question that with these results and others, a prospective randomized trial is ethically justified

Reference

[1] Watson, K; Ballet, F. The SLAC wrsit: scapholunate advanced collapse pattern of degenerative arthritis. *J Hand Surg,* 1984, 9A, 358-365.

[2] Cohen, M; Kozin, S. Degenerative arthritis of the wrist: proximal row carpectomy versus scaphoid exc

[3] Krakauer, J; Bishop, A; Cooney, W. Surgical treatment of scapholunate advanced collapse. *J Hand Surg,* 1994, 19A, 751-759.ision and four-corner arthrodesis. *J Hand Surg,* 2001, 26A, 94-104

[4] Krimmer, H; Lanz, U. Der postraumatische karpale Kollaps. *Der Unfallchirurg,* 2000, 103, 260-266.

[5] Lukas, B; Herter, F; Englert, A; Bäcker, K. Der fortgeschrittene karpale Kollpas: resektion der proximalen Handwurzelreihe oder mediokarpale Teilarthrodese? *Handchir, Mikrochir, Plast Chir,* 2003, 35, 304-309.

[6] Nakamura, R; Horii, E; Watanabe, K; Nakao, E; Kato, H; Tsudnoda, K. Proximal row carpectomy versus limited wrist arthrodesis for advanced Kienbock's disease. *J Hand Surg 1998,* 23B, 741-745.

[7] Tomaino, M; Miller, R; Cole, I; Burton, R. Scapholunate advanced collapse wrist: proximal row carpectomy or limited wrist arthrodesis with scaphoid excision. *J Hand Surg,* 1994; 19A: 134-142.

[8] Vanhove, W; De Vil, J; Van Seymortier, P; Boone, B; Verdonk, R. Proximal row carpectomy versus four corner arthrodesis as a treatment for SLAC (scapholunate advanced collapse) wrist. *J.Hand Surg*., 2008, 33E, 118-125

[9] Wyrick, J; Sern, P; Kiefhaber, T. Motion preserving procedures in the treatment of scapholunate advanced collapse wrist: proximal row carpectomy versus four-corner arthrodesis. *J Hand Surg,* 1995, 20A, 965-970.

[10] Berger, RA; Bishop, AT; Bettinger, PC. New dorsal capsulotomy for the surgical exposure of the wrist. Ann Plast Surg 1995, 35, 54-59

[11] Hudak, P; Amadio, P; Bombardier, C. Development of an upper extremity outcome measure: the DASH. *Am J Indust Med,* 1996, 29, 602-608

[12] De Smet, L; De Kezel, R; Degreef, I; Debeer, P. Responsiveness of the Dutch version of the DASH as an outcome measure for carpal tunnel syndrome. *J Hand Surg,* 2007, 32E, 74-76.

[13] MacDermid, J; Turgeon, T; Richards, R; Beadle, M; Roth, J. Patient rating of wrist pain and disability: a reliable and valid measurement tool. Journal of Orthopaedic Trauma, 1998, 12, 577-586.

[14] Bolano, L; Green, D. Wrist arthrodesis in posttraumatic arthritis: a comparison of 2 methods. *J Hand Surg* 1993, 18A, 786-79.

[15] Field, J; Herbert, J; Prosser, R. Total wrist fusion: a functional assessment. *J Hand Surg* 1996, 21B, 429-43

[16] Hastings, H; Weiss, A; Quenzer, D; Wiedeman, G; Hanington, K; Strickland, J. Arthrodesis of the wrist for post-traumatic disorders. *J Bone Joint Surg* 1996; 78A: 897-902.

[17] Houshian, S; Schrøder, H. Wrist arthrodesis with the AO Titatnium wrist fusion plate: a consecutive series of 42 cases. *J Hand Surg* 2001, 26B, 355-359

[18] Kalb, K; Ludwig, A; Tauscher, A; Landslettner, B; Wiemer, P; Krimmer, H. Behandlungergebnisse nach operativer handgelenkversteifung. *Handchir, Microchir, Plast Chir,* 1999, 31, 253-259.

[19] Leighton, R; Petrie, D. Arthrodesis of the wrist. *Can J Surg* 1987, 30, 115-116.

[20] O'Bierne, J; Boyer, M; Axelrod, T. Wrist arthrodesis using a dynamic compression plate. *J Bone Joint Surg,* 1995, 77B, 700-794.

[21] Sagerman, S; Palmer, A. Wrist arthrodesis using a dynamic compression plate. *J Hand Surg,* 1996, 21B, 437-441

[22] Sauerbier, M; Kluge, S; Bickert, B; Germann, G. Subjective and objective outcomes after total wrist arthrodesis in patients with radiocarpal arthrosis or Kienböck's disease. *Chir Main,* 2000, 19, 223-231.

[23] Shayfer, S; Toledano, B; Ruby, L. Wrist arthrodesis, an alternative technique. *Orthopedics,* 1998, 21, 1139-1143

[24] Weiss A; Hastings H. Wrist arthrodesis for traumatic conditions; a study of plate and local bone graft application. *J Hand Surg* 1995; 20A: 50-56.

[25] Weiss, A; Wiedemaman, G; Quenzers, D; Hanington, K; Hastings, H; Strickland, J. Upper extremity function after wrist arthrodesis. *J Hand Surg,* 1995, 20A, 813-817.

[26] Dap, F. L'arthrodèse du poignet: alternative à la résection de la première rangée des os du carpe. *Ann Chir Main,* 1992, 11, 285-291.

[27] De Smet, L; Truyen, J. Arthrodesis of the wrist for osteoarthritis: outcome with a minimum follow-up of 4 years. *J Hand Surg,* 2003, 28B, 575-57

[28] Gaisne, E; Dap, F; Bour, C; Merle, M. Arthrodèse du poignet chez le travailleur manuel. *Rev Chir Orthop* 1991, 77, 537-544

[29] Nagy, L; Buchler, V. Ist die panarthrodese der Goldstandard der Handgelenkchirurgie? *Handchir, Mikrochir, Plast Chir,* 1998, 30, 291-297

[30] Palmer, A; Werner, F; Murphy, D; Glisson, R. Functional wrist motion: a biomechanical study. *J Hand Surg,* 1985, 10, 39- 46

[31] Blumfield, R; Champoux, J. A biomechanical study of normal functional wrist motion. *Clin Orthop,* 1984, 187, 23-25.

[32] Ryu, J; Cooney, W; Askew, L *et al.* Functional ranges of motion of the wrist joint. *J Hand Surg,* 1991, 202, 12-15.

[33] Nelson, DL. Functional wrist motion. *Hand Clin,* 1997; 13(1), 83-92.

[34] Adams, BD; Grosland, NM; Murphy, DM; McCullough, M. Impact of impaired wrist motion on hand and upper-extremity performance *J Hand Surg [Am]* 2003 ; 28 : 898-890.

[35] De Smet L. Relationship of impairment, disability and working status after reconstructive surgery of the wrist. *Hand Surg,* 2007

[36] Alnot, J; Bleton, R. La résection de la première rangée des os du carpe dans les séquelles des fractures du scaphoide. *Ann Chir Main,* 1992, 11, 269-275.

[37] Begley, B; Engber, W. Proximal row carpectomy in advanced Kienbock's disease. *J Hand Surg* 1994, 19A, 1016-1018.

[38] Crabbe, W. Excision of the proximal row of the carpus. *J Bone Joint Surg,* 1964, 46B, 708-711.

[39] Culp, R; McGuigan, F; Turner, M; Lichtman, D; Osterman, A; McCarrol, H. Proximal row carpectomy: a multicenter study. *J Hand Surg,* 1993, 18A, 19-25

[40] De Smet, L; Robijns, F; Degreef, I. Outcome of proximal row carpectomy. Scandinavian Journal of Plastic and Reconstructive Surgery and Hand Surgery, 2006, 40, 302-306

[41] Didonna, M; Kiefhaber, T; Stein, P. Proximal row carpectomy: study with a minimum of ten years follow-up. *J Bone Joint Surg* 2004, 86A, 2359-2365.

[42] Ferlic, D; Clayton, M; Mills, M. Proximal row carpectomy: review of rheumatoid and nonrheumatoid wrists. *J Hand Surg,* 1991, 16A, 420-424.

[43] Foucher, G; Chmiel, Z. La résection de la première rangée du carpe. A propos d'une série de 21 cas. *Rev Chir Orthop,* 1992, 78, 372-378

[44] Green, D. Proximal row carpectomy. *Hand Clin,* 1987, 3, 163-168.20.

[45] Imbreglia, J; Broudy, A; Hagberg, W; McKernan, D. Proximal row carpectomy: clinical evaluation. *J Hand Surg,* 1990, 15A, 426-430.

[46] Inglis, A; Jones, E. Proximal row carpectomy for diseases of the proximal row. *J Bone Joint Surg,* 1977, 59A, 460-463

[47] Inoue, G; Miura, T. Proximal row carpectomy in perilunate dislocations and lunatomalacia. *Act Orthop Scand,* 1990, 61, 449-452.

[48] Jebson, P; Hayes, E; Engber, W. Proximal row carpectomy: a minimum 10-year follow-up study. *J Hand Surg,* 2003, 28A, 561-569.

[49] Jorgensen, E. Proximal row carpectomy. An end result study of twenty-two casis. *J Bone Joint Surg,* 1969, 51A, 1104-1111

[50] Legre, R; Sassoon, D. Etude multicentrique de 143 cas de résection de la première rangée des os du carpe. *Ann Chir Main,* 1992, 11, 237-263.

[51] Luchetti, R; Soragni, O; Fairplay, T. Proximal row carpectomy through a palmar approach. *J Hand Surg,* 1998, 23B: 406-409.

[52] Nagelvoort, R; Kon, M, Schuurman, A. Proximal row carpectomy: a worthwhile salvage procedure. *Scand J Plast Reconstr Surg Hand Surg,* 2002, 36, 289-299.

[53] Neviaser, R. Proximal row carpectomy for posttraumatic disorders of the carpus. *J Hand Surg,* 1983, 8, 301-305.

[54] Neviaser, R. On resection of the proximal row. *Clin Orthop,* 1986, 202, 12-15.

[55] Rettig, M; Raskin, K. Long-term assessment of proximal row carpectomy for chronic perilunate dislocations. *J Hand Surg* 1999, 24A, 1231-1236

[56] Salomon, G; Eaton, R. Proximal row carpectomy with partial capitate resection. *J Hand Surg,* 1996, 21A, 2-8

[57] Schernberg, G; Lamarque, B; Genevray, J; Gerard, Y. La résection arthroplastique de la première rangée des os du carpe. *Ann Chir,* 1981, 35, 269-274.49

[58] Steenwerckx, A; De Smet, L; Zachee, B; Fabry, G. Proximal row carpectomy: an alternative to wrist arthrodesis. *Act Orthop Belg,* 1997, 63, 1-7.

[59] Streich, N; Martini, A; Daeke, W. Resektion der proximalen Handwurzelreihe bei karpalen Kollaps. *Handchir Mikrochir Plast Chir,* 2003, 35, 299-303.

[60] Tomaino, M; Delsignore, J; Burton, R. Long-term results following proximal row carpectomy. *J Hand Surg,* 1994, 19A, 694-703.

[61] Tränkle, M; Sauerbier, M; Blum, K; Bickert, B; Germann, G. Die Entfernung der proximalen Handwurzelreihe als bewegungserhaltender Eingriff beim karpalen Kollpas. *Unfallchirurg,* 2003, 106, 1010-1015.

[62] Voche, Ph, Merle, M. L'arthrodèse des 4 os du poignet. *Rev Chir Orthop,* 1993, 79, 456-463.

[63] Welby, F; Alnot, J. La résection de la première rangée du carpe: poignet post-traumatique et maladie de Kienbock. *Chir Main,* 2003, 22, 148-153.

[64] Ashmead, D; Watson, K; Damon, C; Herber, S; Paly, W. Scapholunate advanced collpase wrist salvage. *J Hand Surg,* 1994, 19A, 741-750.

[65] Bertrand, M; Coulet, B; Chammas, M; Rigout, C ; Allieu, Y. L'arthrodèse des quatre os du poignet. *Rev Chir Orthop,* 2002, 88, 286-292.5.

[66] Dagregorio, G; Saint Cast, Y; Fouque, P. L'influence de l'angle de fusion capitolunaire sur le résultat fonctionnel de l'intervention de Watson réalisée dans 58 cas de collapsus carpiens avancés. *La Main,* 1998, 3, 363-373.

[67] Garcia-Lopez, A; Perez-Ubeda, J; Marco, F; Molina, M; Lopez-Duran, L. A modified technique for four-bone fusion for advanced carpal collapse (SLAC/SNAC wrist). *J Hand Surg,* 2001, 26B, 352-354.

[68] Gill, D; Ireland, D. Limmited wrist arthrodesis for the salvage of SLAC wrist. *J Hand Surg,* 1997, 22B, 461- 465

[69] .Kadji, O; Duteille, F; Dautel, G; Merle, M. Arthrodèse carpiene des quatre os versus arthrodèse capitolunaire. A propos de 40 patients. *Chir Main,* 2002, 21, 5-12.

[70] Kirschenbaum, D; Schnieder, L; Kirkpatrick, W; Adams, D; Cody, R. Scaphoid excision and capitolunate arthrodesis for radioscaphoid arthritis. *J Hand Surg,* 1993; 18A, 780-785

[71] Sauerbier, M; Trankle, M.; Linsner, G; Bickert, B; Germann, G. Midcarpal arthrodesis with scaphoid excision and interposition bone graft in the treatment of advanced carpal collapse (SLAC/SNAC wrist): operative technique and outcome assessment. *J Hand Surg,* 2000, 25B, 341-345.

In: Hand Surgery: Preoperative Expectations...
Editor: Robert H. Beckingsworth
ISBN: 978-1-60876-280-4

Chapter 6

Ulnar-Sided Wrist Pathology, Evaluation and an Extraarticular Cause of Impingement

***Kirtie Lo*[1]*, Lois Carlson* [1] *and Ronit Wollstein*[2]**
[1]The Hand Center, 85 Seymour Street, Suite 816, Hartford, CT 06106
[2]Division of Plastic Surgery, University of Pittsburgh, 200 Lothrop Street, Pittsburgh, PA 15213-2582, USA

Abstract

Pain in the area of the ulnar wrist remains a diagnostic and therapeutic challenge for the hand surgeon. Better delineation of the possible etiologies of ulnar wrist pain and correlation with their clinical, arthroscopic, and radiographic findings is critical to enhancing our ability to treat these patients. The authors suggest a primary distinction between intraarticular pathology (in the ulnocarpal joint) and extraarticular pathology. This organization provides the basis for the algorithmic approach presented in this chapter.

Intraarticular causes include TFCC tears, ulnar impaction, and lunotriquetral tears Extraarticular causes encompass ulnar styloid triquetral impaction, ulnar impingement, DRUJ arthritis, pisotriquetral joint dysfunction, hamate and triquetral fractures, and ECU disorders. A novel extraarticular cause of ulnar-sided wrist pain, Triquetral Impingement Ligament Tear (TILT) syndrome, is presented. Each of these causes has specific symptoms and findings on physical and radiographic exam. Arthroscopy is useful for diagnosis and treatment of intraarticular problems, and can confirm isolated extraarticular disease when intraarticular findings are normal. The algorithm presented in this chapter aids the clinician in making the correct diagnosis and choosing the appropriate treatment.

Introduction

Ulnar-sided wrist pain remains a diagnostic challenge for the treating surgeon. Though treatment algorithms have been suggested, the diagnosis is often not readily apparent on clinical exam, and further testing is needed.[1] Even with positive test results, many cases of ulnar sided wrist pain remain obscure and therefore difficult to treat. A better understanding and description of the different pathologies causing ulnar wrist pain and correlation with their clinical, arthroscopic, and radiographic findings is essential in improving our ability to diagnose and treat these patients. The diagnosis of a triangular fibrocartilage complex (TFCC) tear does not always provide the clinical solution, especially since the anatomy of the TFCC itself is complex and unclear, encompassing more than one joint. It has become increasingly evident that an extraarticular group of pathologies also causes ulnar-sided wrist pain. [2-7] We believe that it is helpful to approach the ulnar side of the wrist with an initial distinction between pathologies that are intraarticular (ulnocarpal) and extraarticular.

Anatomy

The ulnar aspect of the wrist is bounded by tendons and ligaments that blend together into a uniform mass.[8] Much of the support is from the volar radiocarpal ligaments. This support is transmitted via the TFCC and annular disk from their strong dorsal, radial attachments to the volar ulnolunate and ulnotriquetral ligaments, which are the volar floor of the TFCC complex.[8,9] The lunotriquetral joint forms the distal portion of the ulnocarpal joint and is intracapsular.The dorsal ligaments of the ulnar wrist are weaker stabilizers of the ulnar side of the wrist. The dorsal wrist capsule is reinforced by the extrinsic radiocarpal ligament, which arises from the radius and passes distally and ulnarly, where it inserts into the lunate and triquetrum. This is part of the dorsal V shaped ligaments described by Viegas et al. [10This ligament, along with the floor of the sixth extensor compartment, forms the dorsal attachments of the TFCC and prevents volar subluxation of the ulnar carpus. The ulnar collateral ligament has been described as a thickening of the wrist capsule and extends from the base of the ulnar styloid to the triquetrum. It is not clear whether this structure exists. The extensor retinaculum overlies and fuses with these structures.[8,9]

Intraarticular Ulnar Sided Wrist Pathology-TFCC Tears

Much of the literature has concentrated on the intraarticular (ulnocarpal) component of ulnar sided wrist pain.[11-13] Arthroscopy has greatly enhanced our understanding of the ulnar side of the wrist and is, at this time, the gold standard for ulnar wrist diagnosis in general [11, 14-16] and for the diagnosis of TFCC tear more specifically.

The diagnosis of a TFCC tear is made based on the clinical presentation, imaging, and arthroscopy. The history often includes a distinct traumatic incident to the wrist. Patients complain of pain localized to the ulnar side of the wrist. Clicking or snapping can accompany the pain, especially with tasks requiring gripping or forearm rotation. Tenderness and swelling are usually present around the anatomic area of the radiocarpal portion of the TFCC, ulnar carpus and distal radio-ulnar joint (DRUJ). Treatment is based on Palmer's classification scheme, with class 1 involving traumatic injuries to the TFCC and class 2 including degenerative damage and tears. Class 2 injuries therefore encompass the damage sustained with ulnar impaction into the carpus.

Class 1 and 2 are further subdivided with specific treatments for each subclass. Class 1A refers to isolated central tears without any instability. These can be treated conservatively with immobilization or arthroscopically with debridement. Class 1B lesions are peripheral tears at the base of the ulnar styloid. These avulse off the distal ulna with or without a fracture of the ulna styloid. Acutely, these also can be treated with immobilization. More chronic lesions may require arthroscopic or open repair addressing any ulnar styloid fragment that may be present. Class 1C encompasses traumatic disruptions of the ulnolunate or ulnotriquetral ligaments of the TFCC. These lesions require repair plus capsulodesis or repair of the extrinsic ligaments. Class 1D are disruptions from the sigmoid notch of the radius and can be treated with re-attachment to the sigmoid notch.

Class 2 lesions, often a result of chronic load to the ulnar side of the wrist, are classified according to the location and severity of the disease. Class 2A is only mild chrondromalacia of the articular disc without perforation. Class 2B is wearing of the TFCC with chrondromalacia of the ulnar head and/or lunate. Starting with class 2C, we start to see true perforations of the TFCC. Class 2D and 2E involve lunotriquetral ligament disruption with 2E representing end-stage arthritis of the ulnar carpus and DRUJ. Class 2 lesions can be treated conservatively using immobilization, nonsteroidal anti-inflammatory medication, cortisone injections, and activity modification. Surgical options for the more advance classes include debridement, ulnar shortening, partial or complete ulnar head excision, and interposition arthroplasty.[17 18]

Ulnar impaction syndrome, ulnocarpal abutment syndrome, or ulnocarpal impaction (UCI) all refer to abnormal contact load between the ulna and carpus. In ulnar impaction, the long ulna impacts into the carpus, usually involving the lunate and lunotriquetral joint and rarely the triquetrum. Ulnar impaction is a separate entity from ulnar impingement, in which the shortened ulna impinges into the radius causing extraarticular pathology. [19]

Clinically, patients with ulnar impaction present with insidious onset of ulnar-sided wrist pain that is increased with pronation and ulnar deviation. The fovea sign [20is positive and ulnar-positive variance is usually present. Subchondral sclerosis, subchondral cysts, and "kissing" lesions of the lunate, triquetrum, and ulnar head are seen on standard radiographs. Conservative treatment such as intermittent immobilization, nonsteroidal anti-inflammatory drugs, avoidance of ulnar-deviation maneuvers, and corticosteroid injections can be tried initially. Surgical options include ulnar-shortening osteotomy and open or arthroscopic wafer procedure.[18]

Lunotriquetral ligament tears secondary to ulnar impaction or other causes (acutely with a hyperextension or twisting injury) can also cause ulnar sided wrist pain. These patients will have positive LT ballottement and shuck tests. The LT ballottement test is performed with the lunate fixed by one hand while the other hand applies a dorsal and palmar force across the LT joint. The shuck test is performed with the thumb over the pisiform and fingers over the LT joint. If there is LT instability, clicking or pain occurs as the wrist is taken through active and passive radial and ulnar deviation. Acutely, LT ligament sprains or tears can be treated in a cast for 4-6 weeks. Chronic tears or injuries that fail conservative treatment can be managed arthroscopically with debridement if sufficiently stable. With the development of arthritis in this joint, however, LT fusion is necessary.[21,22]

Extraarticular Ulnar Sided Wrist Pathology

It has become increasingly clear that an extraarticular group of pathologies also cause ulnar sided wrist pain. This heterogeneous group includes diagnoses that have not always been adequately addressed clinically or extensively studied. An entity distinct from the classic ulnocarpal impaction syndrome called ulnar styloid triquetral impaction has also been described. This is an abnormal contact between the ulnar styloid and triquetrum, which results in extraarticular pain and point tenderness directly over the ulnar styloid instead of the lunate. The provocative test is rotating the wrist from pronation to full supination while maintaining the wrist in dorsiflexion. Radiographs can reveal a decreased distance between the ulnar styloid and triquetrum when compared to the other side. The diagnosis can be confirmed by injecting lidocaine directly over the tip of the ulnar styloid. Treatment starts with conservative measures and can progress to ulnar styloid excision. If the diagnosis is complicated by another diagnosis, such as classic ulnocarpal impaction syndrome, then both entities will have to be addressed surgically. [5]

Ulnar impingement syndrome is usually iatrogenic following distal ulnar resection, but can also be due to growth arrest of the ulnar epiphysis or congenital abnormalities. The shortened ulna impinges on the radius, causing pain and crepitus in the distal radioulnar joint (DRUJ) with pronation and supination. Forearm rotation can be limited and grip is often weak. X-rays demonstrate scalloping of the distal radius due to the impinging distal ulna. Treatment includes various techniques that attempt to restore stability to the distal ulna, including ulnar lengthening and procedures using the ECU, FCU, and soft tissue interposition.[19

Also causing ulnar- sided wrist pain is DRUJ arthritis, which can be a consequence of trauma or systemic disorders such as rheumatoid arthritis. Symptoms are similar to ulnar impingement syndrome with pain, clicking, weak grip, and decreased range of motion. Radiographs will show joint narrowing and osteophyte formation. CT scans and arthroscopy can further delineate the pathology. Nonsteroidals, cortisone injection, and activity modification can be beneficial, but prolonged immobilization will only increase stiffness. Surgical options include treating the underlying pathology, for example a malunited distal radius fracture, if the arthritis is mild. As arthritic changes worsen, surgery consists of distal ulna resection, hemiresection with or without interposition, and matched ulna arthroplasty as well as joint replacement or ulnar head replacement. [23,24 25-27]

One volar extraarticular cause of ulnar sided wrist pain is pisotriquetral joint dysfunction, including fractures of the pisiform or arthritis of the joint. The pisiform is a sesamoid bone within the flexor carpi ulnaris (FCU) tendon and articulates with the triquetrum. It is therefore questionable whether this joint actually is involved in the biomechanics of the wrist joint or whether it belongs to the wrist at all. Pain, however, is localized to the volar hypothenar region of the hand, and provocative maneuvers such as the pisotriquetral (PT) grind and apprehension test will be positive[28]. In the differential diagnosis of pain in the hypothenar area, the contents of Guyon's canal should be considered (ulnar nerve symptoms or ulnar artery vascular pathology). Diagnosis can be established with a carpal tunnel radiographic view, or 30° supination view. Confirmation of the diagnosis can be made with a local lidocaine injection into the PT joint. Treatment initially consists of splinting, nonsteroidal anti-inflammatory medications (NSAIDS), and cortisone injections. Fractures can be treated with a short arm cast immobilizing the hand in slight ulnar deviation and palmar flexion for 6 weeks. If conservative measures fail, the pisiform can be excised without sacrificing significant function. [29]

Hamate fractures can also cause extraarticular ulnar sided wrist pain. Hamate fractures usually result from a direct blow to the hypothenar eminence or an axial blow with a clenched fist. Pain, swelling, and ecchymosis on the ulnar border with point tenderness over the hamate can indicate a hamate fracture. The diagnosis can be confirmed with radiographs and a computerized tomography (CT) scan if an occult fracture or fracture-dislocation is suspected. These fractures are often missed, but should be suspected with traumatic dislocations of the ring and small finger carpometacarpal joints.

Acute fractures of the hook of the hamate can be treated with a short arm cast. Similarly, acute fractures of the body if minimally displaced and stable can also be treated conservatively. Fractures with joint subluxation or intraarticular displacement, however, require surgical treatment, usually involving reduction and fixation with wires or mini fragment screws. Hamate hook fractures that fail conservative treatment or are not diagnosed in the posttraumatic period may fail to unite and will then require excision of the fragment and release of Guyon's canal. [30]

In addition to fractures of the hamate, fractures of the triquetrum also present as ulnar sided wrist pain. These can result from a fall on an outstretched hand with a dorsiflexed wrist. Pain, swelling, tenderness, and ecchymosis over the dorsum of the triquetrum are usually present. Standard radiographs can demonstrate the fracture, especially if an oblique 30° of pronation view is included. CT scans should also be obtained if radiographs are negative but a high degree of suspicion remains. Treatment of isolated triquetrum fractures is 6 weeks of immobilization in a short arm cast. These fractures, however, are often associated with other more extensive injuries, such as a transtriquetral peri-lunate dislocation, which require immediate treatment. Triquetrohamate arthrosis has also been described as causing ulnar wrist pain [31]

In addition to bony abnormalities, pathology of the extensor carpi ulnaris (ECU) such as subluxation and stenosing tenosynovitis can also lead to ulnar sided wrist pain. ECU subluxation presents as painful snapping on the dorsal-ulnar border of the wrist. Clinical exam demonstrates gross instability of the tendon. Standard radiographs are usually normal, but MRI can show the subluxation. Although most acute injuries are treated surgically with reconstruction of the tendon sheath, these injuries could also be treated conservatively in a long arm cast. [32]

ECU stenosing tendonitis presents with pain, swelling, and tenderness along the ECU tendon and thus, can be easily confused with subluxation of the tendon. Symptoms, however, will be relieved by lidocaine injection into the tendon subsheath. Immobilization, activity modification, nonsteroidals, and cortisone injection are all reasonable nonoperative treatment options. For failure of conservative measures, surgical release of the sixth dorsal compartment can be effective as long as the ulnar subsheath is not released and the extensor retinaculum is closed. These measures will prevent ECU subluxation. [33]

In 1999, Watson et al. described a novel cause of extraarticular ulnar sided wrist pain, Triquetral Impingement Ligament Tear (TILT) syndrome. [34-36] Patients presented with ulnar-sided wrist pain and swelling, and a decrease in wrist range of motion (ROM) and grip strength. On examination, there was point tenderness with palpation over the dorsal ulnar aspect of the triquetral bone. The exact nature of the impinging tissue remains unclear, though it was originally described as the "ulnar sling mechanism".[34] The impingement is caused by a redundant, free soft tissue mass impinging on the dorsal triquetrum, leading to inflammation and erosion of the triquetrum with chondromalacia. Direct visualization of the ulnar carpal bones during surgery showed evidence of hyperemic bone often with exposed subchondral bone with a soft spongy cortex.[34]

In an unpublished series, 14 consecutive patients with the clinical picture of TILT were evaluated prior to surgery. All patients had MRI's performed and 7 patients had an arthroscopy done. MRI demonstrated evidence of focal subchondral edema in the triquetrum and cystic changes in the triquetrum. Of the patients undergoing arthroscopy, two patients had evidence of some radial sided degeneration with minimal synovitis. The ulnar side of the wrist was found to be normal in all arthroscopies.

The weak dorsal ligamentous structures of the wrist are probably torn in this syndrome by an injury. The redundant tissue then creates a physical impediment to motion and causes pain by compressing chronically inflamed tissue. In 13 out of the 14 patients at surgery, we found synovium or loose connective tissue in the dorsal aspect of the wrist, and in one patient, an osteochondral fracture/flap was present that was treated with debridement. The treatment consists of surgical removal of the inflamed "impinging" tissue.

Conclusions

The ulnar side of the wrist remains a diagnostic challenge. The anatomy has not been clearly defined, and our clinical tests are often insufficient to diagnose the problem. Other tests, such as MRI, do not reliably identify pathology that is clinically relevant. To assist in the clinical diagnosis, we have divided the known pathologies into intraarticular (ulnocarpal joint) and extraarticular problems (see flow chart).

The intraarticular pathology consists mostly of tears of the TFCC and other intraarticular ligaments such as the ulnotriquetral or lunotriquetral ligaments. These can be best visualized, diagnosed, and often treated through arthroscopy. The group of extraarticular ulnar wrist pathologies includes an assorted, ill defined and poorly studied group of pathologies. These can include the DRUJ, the dorsal hamate or triquetrum, and the ECU, and cannot be visualized through arthroscopy but can be differentiated based on the location and character of the pain. This diagnostic algorithm may assist in the approach to what is still the "black box" of the wrist.

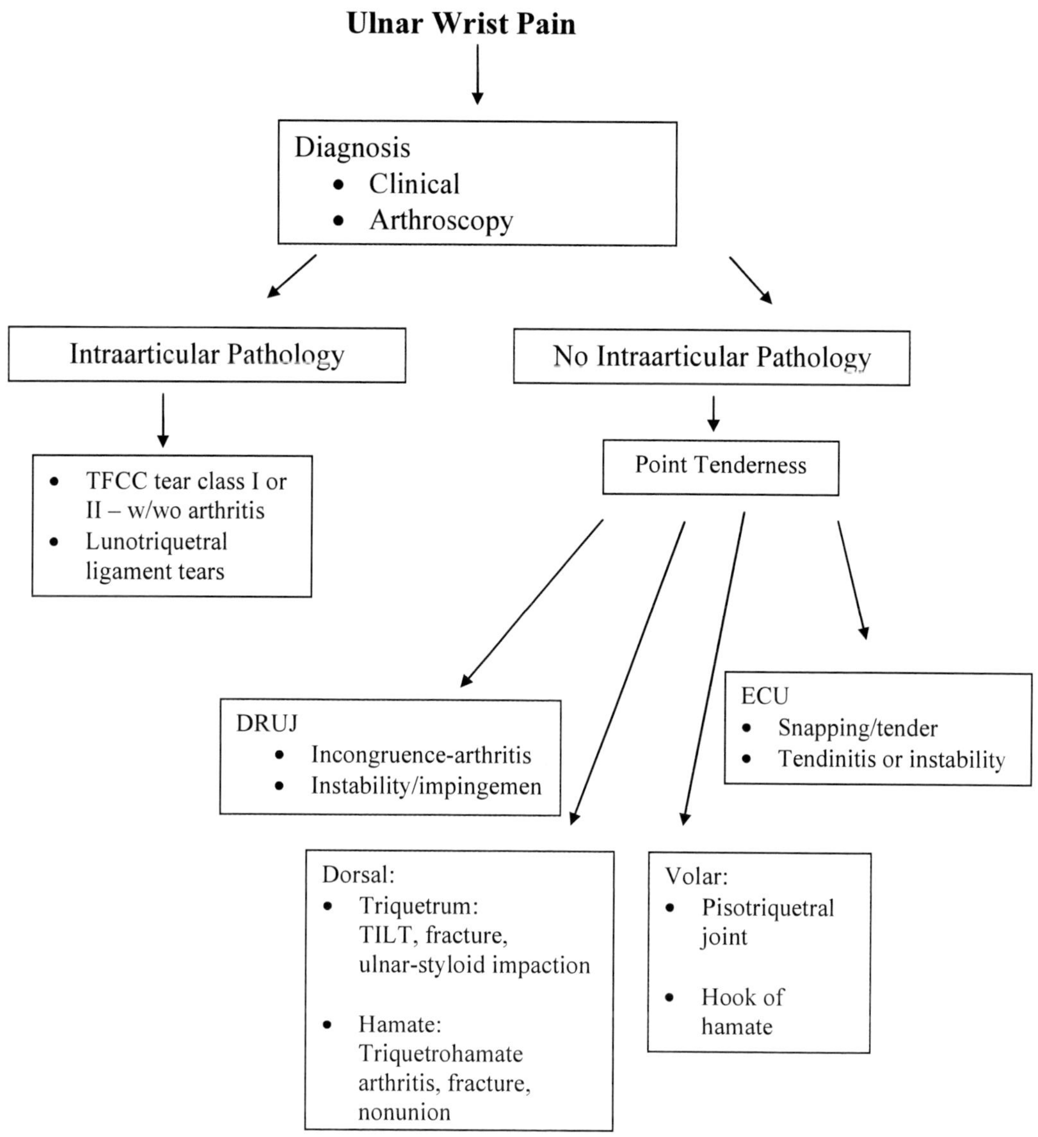

References

[1] Stanley, JK; Hodgson, SP; Royle, SG. An approach to the diagnosis of chronic wrist pain. *Ann Chir Main Memb Super*, 1994, 13, 202-205.

[2] Bain, GI; Bidwell, TA. Arthroscopic excision of ulnar styloid in stylocarpal impaction. *Arthroscopy*, 2006, 22, 677 e671-673.

[3] Bottke, CA; Louis, DS; Braunstein, EM. Diagnosis and treatment of obscure ulnar sided wrist pain. *Orthopedics*, 1989, 12, 1075-1079.

[4] Crimmins, CA; Jones, NF. Stenosing tenosynovitis of the extensor carpi ulnaris. *Ann Plast Surg*, 1995, 35, 105-107.

[5] Giachino, AA; McIntyre, AI; Guy, KJ; Conway, AF. Ulnar styloid triquetral impaction. *Hand Surg*, 2007, 12, 123-134.

[6] Bhatia, A; Pisoh, T; Touam, C; Oberlin, C. Incidence and distribution of scaphotrapezotrapezoidal arthritis in 73 fresh cadaveric wrists. *Ann Chir Main Memb Super*, 1996, 15, 220-225.

[7] Dharap, AS; Al-Hashimi, H; Kassab, S; Abu-Hijleh, MF. The hamate facet of the lunate: a radiographic study in an Arab population from Bahrain. *Surg Radiol Anat*, 2006, 28, 185-188.

[8] Taleisnik, J. The ligaments of the wrist. *J Hand Surg* [Am], 1976, 1, 110-118.

[9] Palmer, AK; Werner, FW. The triangular fibrocartilage complex of the wrist--anatomy and function. *J Hand Surg* [Am], 1981, 6, 153-162.

[10] Viegas, SF. The dorsal ligaments of the wrist. *Hand Clin*, 2001, 17, 65-75, vi.

[11] Baehser-Griffith, P; Bednar, JM; Osterman, AL; Culp, R. Arthroscopic repairs of triangular fibrocartilage complex tears. Aorn J 1997, 66, 101-102, 105-111, quiz 112, 115, 117-108.

[12] Bohringer, G; Schadel-Hopfner, M; Petermann, J; Gotzen, L. A method for all-inside arthroscopic repair of Palmer 1B triangular fibrocartilage complex tears. Arthroscopy 2002, 18, 211-213.

[13] Lubiatowski, P; Romanowski, L; Splawski, R; Manikowski, W; Ogrodowicz, P. Treatment of injury of the triangular fibrocartilage complex (TFCC). *Ortop Traumatol Rehabil*, 2006, 8, 256-262.

[14] Weiss, LE; Taras, JS; Sweet, S; Osterman, AL. Lunotriquetral injuries in the athlete. Hand Clin 2000, 16, 433-438.

[15] Yao, J; Dantuluri, P; Osterman, AL. A novel technique of all-inside arthroscopic triangular fibrocartilage complex repair. *Arthroscopy*, 2007, 23, 1357 e1351-1354.

[16] Bednar JM, Osterman AL. The role of arthroscopy in the treatment of traumatic triangular fibrocartilage injuries. *Hand Clin*, 1994, 10, 605-614.

[17] Palmer, AK. Triangular fibrocartilage complex lesions: a classification. *J Hand Surg* [Am], 1989, 14, 594-606.

[18] Sachar, K. Ulnar-sided wrist pain: evaluation and treatment of triangular fibrocartilage complex tears, ulnocarpal impaction syndrome, and lunotriquetral ligament tears. *J Hand Surg* [Am], 2008, 33, 1669-1679.

[19] Bell, MJ; Hill, RJ; McMurtry, RY. Ulnar impingement syndrome. *J Bone Joint Surg Br,* 1985, 67, 126-129.

[20] Tay, SC; Tomita, K; Berger, RA. The "ulnar fovea sign" for defining ulnar wrist pain: an analysis of sensitivity and specificity. *J Hand Surg* [Am], 2007, 32, 438-444.

[21] Guidera, PM; Watson, HK; Dwyer, TA; Orlando, G; Zeppieri, J; Yasuda, M. Lunotriquetral arthrodesis using cancellous bone graft. J Hand Surg [Am] 2001, 26, 422-427.

[22] Pin, PG; Young, VL; Gilula, LA; Weeks, PM. Management of chronic lunotriquetral ligament tears. *J Hand Surg* [Am], 1989, 14, 77-83.

[23] Bowers, WH. Distal radioulnar joint arthroplasty. Current concepts. *Clin Orthop Relat Res*, 1992, 104-109.

[24] Watson, HK; Ryu, JY; Burgess, RC. Matched distal ulnar resection. *J Hand Surg* [Am], 1986, 11, 812-817.

[25] Herzberg, G. Management of bilateral advanced rheumatoid wrist destruction. *J Hand Surg* [Am], 2008, 33, 1192-1195.

[26] Scheker, LR. Implant arthroplasty for the distal radioulnar joint. J Hand Surg [Am] 2008, 33, 1639-1644.

[27] Kopylov, P; Tagil, M. Distal radioulnar joint replacement. Tech Hand Up Extrem Surg 2007, 11, 109-114.

[28] Rayan, GM. Pisiform ligament complex syndrome and pisotriquetral arthrosis. *Hand Clin*, 2005, 21, 507-517.

[29] Carroll, RE; Coyle, MP; Jr. Dysfunction of the pisotriquetral joint: treatment by excision of the pisiform. *J Hand Surg* [Am], 1985, 10, 703-707.

[30] Whalen, JL; Bishop, AT; Linscheid, RL. Nonoperative treatment of acute hamate hook fractures. *J Hand Surg* [Am], 1992, 17, 507-511.

[31] Yao, J; Osterman, AL. Arthroscopic techniques for wrist arthritis (radial styloidectomy and proximal pole hamate excisions). *Hand Clin*, 2005, 21, 519-526.

[32] Rowland, SA; Acute traumatic subluxation of the extensor carpi ulnaris tendon at the wrist. *J Hand Surg* [Am], 1986, 11, 809-811.

[33] Hajj, AA; Wood, MB. Stenosing tenosynovitis of the extensor carpi ulnaris. *J Hand Surg* [Am], 1986, 11, 519-520.

[34] Watson, HK; Weinzweig, J. Triquetral impingement ligament tear (tilt). *J Hand Surg* [Br], 1999, 24, 321-324.

[35] Gross, SC; Watson, HK; Strickland, JW; Palmer, AK; Brenner, LH; Fatti, J. Triquetral-lunate arthritis secondary to synostosis. *J Hand Surg* [Am] 1989, 14, 95-102.

[36] Kao, SD; Watson, HK; Fong, D. Congenital triquetral absence: a case report of an asymptomatic wrist. *J Hand Surg* [Am], 1996, 21, 314-316.

In: Hand Surgery: Preoperative Expectations...
Editor: Robert H. Beckingsworth
ISBN: 978-1-60876-280-4

Chapter 7

An Injectable Mixture of Calcium Phosphate and Calcium Sulfate Cement as an Adjunct to Internal Fixation for Comminuted Distal Radius Fractures

Mario G. Solari and Ronit Wollstein
Department of Surgery, Division of Plastic and Reconstructive Surgery,
University of Pittsburgh, Pittsburgh PA, USA

Abstract

Introduction

Distal radius fracture alignment and stabilization can be a surgical challenge in the face of severe comminution and bone loss. The current standard of care for such cases calls for autologous bone grafting and rigid fixation. In this chapter, we describe a technique using HydroSet (Stryker), a calcium phosphate bone cement, as an adjunct to internal fixation. The technique eliminates the need for autologous bone grafting and the associated donor site morbidity. This bone graft substitute is biocompatible, osteoconductive, and sets quickly with an isothermic reaction. Available bone cements, studies involving the use of bone cement for distal radius fractures, indications, and surgical technique will be reviewed.

Methods

All consecutive severely comminuted distal radius fractures treated by the senior author over a period of 9 months using standard surgical technique and rigid fixation were reviewed. Six females and seven males with an average age of 50.7 (+/-15.9) met criteria. HydroSet bone cement was used in 14 fractures in 14 patients. Radiographs were used to assess healing.

Results

Bony healing was achieved in all but one patient. Severe dorsal comminution with loss of articular surface and articular support was present in 9 cases. In all of these cases HydroSet was used to reconstruct the dorsal articular surface. In one case, the HydroSet was used to reconstruct over 80% of the articular surface. Screws were not drilled into the HydroSet. No collapse was seen on radiographs at 6 weeks follow-up.

Discussion

Bioactive bone cements hold great promise for the treatment of comminuted distal radius fractures. In our case series the use of bone cement eliminated the need for primary autologous bone grafting. It allowed for easier reduction and retention of reduction at the time of surgery due to the quick hardening time. The graft did not allow for screw insertion, and therefore the hardware was used as a buttress for the graft. As there usually was no cavity bound on three sides by bone, post-operative X-rays are full of visible bone graft and are difficult to interpret. However, radial length was maintained 6 weeks postoperatively. Despite limited follow up, the clinical results using HydroSet bone cement are encouraging.

Introduction

Highly comminuted, intra-articular distal radius fractures are a particularly challenging subset of wrist fractures to manage. This fracture type is seen with high-energy trauma and in elderly patients with osteoporotic bone. Loss of bone stock, small fracture fragments, and joint surface incongruity contribute to chronic pain, stiffness, and arthritis.

Closed reduction and cast immobilization has largely been replaced by operative interventions due to the instability of these fractures [1, 2]. External fixation has been a common treatment modality that has yielded improved outcomes over cast immobilization alone. There are, however, well-established limitations of external fixation including the inability to reduce and maintain articular fragments and the disadvantages of prolonged immobilization [3, 4]. Recent advances in plate technology, the understanding of wrist kinematics, and fracture outcome studies, have popularized the use of internal fixation, particularly volar locking plates. While plates can restore both extra-articular parameters and articular congruity, small fracture fragments and crushed cancellous bone can compromise stability. Autologous bone grafting has been used traditionally to fill the metaphyseal void. This has several shortcomings including donor site morbidity and a lack of immediate support to surrounding fragments. One means of addressing this issue is bone cement. Bone cement can be used as a metaphyseal bone substitute and lend support to overlying articular fragments. It can also be used to hold fragments too small to be fixated by hardware.

In this chapter, we discuss available bone cements, review the literature on the use of cements for distal radius fractures, and describe indications and surgical techniques. We describe our preliminary experience using HydroSet (Stryker), a mixture of calcium phosphate and sulfate bone cement, as an adjunct to internal fixation. The technique eliminates the need for autologous bone grafting and the associated donor site morbidity. The support it lends to fragment retention may also allow for less invasive fixation techniques or earlier rehabilitation.

Bone Cements

Polymethyl Methacrylate

An Ideal bone substitute is biocompatible, osteoinductive, osteoconductive, malleable, mechanically strong, resorbable (at a rate in line with new bone formation) and has an appropriate hardening time. The classic bone cement is polymethyl methacrylate (PMMA), an acrylic cement, that has been used successfully to anchor artificial joints. PMMA improves fracture stability in osteoporotic bone [5, 6], and has been used in the treatment of distal radius fractures. Scmalholz et al. [7, 8] successfully used PMMA for non-comminuted, extra-articular re-dislocated distal radius fractures. They found that all treated fractures were healed two years postoperative with the cement surrounded by cortical bone. However, it has several shortcomings that have limited its use for comminuted distal radius fractures. The setting reaction is exothermic which can potentially inhibit fracture healing and injure already traumatized soft tissue. It also shrinks during this process. It is neither resorbable nor incorporated into bone and is difficult to remove.

Calcium Phosphate

The shortcomings of PMMA have sparked research with new materials for fracture management. Calcium phosphate cements are a popular biodegradable alternative. In an attempt to create a cement that is strong enough to allow for short-term stability of the construct, is easy to handle, and can be used to change the position of fragments intraoperatively, different mixtures of calcium phosphate and calcium sulfate have been attempted [9]. Calcium phosphate hardens quickly and takes longer to be replaced by bone, while calcium sulfate is softer and more readily ossified. There are many available commercial formulations of calcium phosphate/sulphate cements giving some variations in properties. In general, they are injectable or malleable putties, osteoconductive, set at body temperature, offer some structural support, and are remodeled. Products that have been used for distal radius fractures include Norian SRS (Synthes), Bonesource (Stryker), and Hydroset (Stryker).

Early cadaveric biomechanical studies testing calcium phosphate cements in distal radius fractures were encouraging. Yetkinler et al., [10] compared four K-wires with Norian SRS alone in cadaveric intra-articular distal radius fractures. Dynamic testing revealed significantly more settling and a larger volar step-off in the K wire group. The ultimate strength was not different between the two groups. Higgins et al. [11], on the other hand, found that Norian SRS when used alone was insufficient to withstand physiologic forces. When used to supplement K-wires, it provided more stable fixation than K-wires alone.

Multiple clinical studies have been performed using calcium phosphate cements for distal radius fractures of varying severity and with different types of hardware. Sanchez-Sotelo et al.[12] evaluated 110 patients with AO A3 or C2 fractures. Half received closed reduction and cast immobilization for 6 weeks or closed reduction, gap debridement through a small incision, and injection of Norian SRS. Improved recovery of range of motion seen in the cement group diminished over time. There were over twice as many cases of malunion in the control group. Kopylov et al.[13] studied forty patients in two groups with redisplaced distal radius fractures. After reduction, fractures were either stabilized with external fixation for five weeks or treated with the injection of Norian SRS and cast immobilization for two weeks. Patients treated with SRS had slightly better grip strength, wrist extension, and forearm supination at seven weeks, however there was no difference in functional parameters at three months or later. The early improvement was due to the earlier mobilization time. Both groups showed a progressive loss of reduction, with the SRS group having significantly worse ulnar variance. Jeyamet al.[14] compared closed reduction and K-wire fixation of Melone type I or IIa fractures in nine patients compared with closed reduction, debridement through a small dorsal incision, and filling of the bone void with Bonesource in a second group of nine patients. All radiologic parameters were worse at 12 and 26 weeks in the Bonesource group as well as grip strength and palmar flexion.

These studies suggest that when calcium phosphate cement is used alone, fracture stability is inadequate. Though treatment with cement may give better results than closed reduction and immobilization alone, many surgeons would consider this "conservative treatment" inadequate for unstable fractures.

In a larger prospective, randomized trial Cassidy et al. treated distal radius fractures with Norian SRS cement alone or with K wires and immobilized for 2 weeks. Controls were immobilized with a cast or external fixator for 6-8 weeks. Functional outcome was better at 6-8 weeks in the cement group, since the controls were immobilized during that entire period. This difference was lost when evaluated at one year. Despite equivalent long-term function, radiographs in the cement only group lost more radial length compared to controls. Fractures requiring K wire fixation in both the control and cement groups had a significantly higher rate of reduction maintenance compared to the groups without K wires. Though the presence of K wires did not influence the overall outcome, cement clearly did not resist all stress forces. Though biomechanical studies[10] demonstrated good compressive strength, low tension and sheer strength may have contributed to loss of reduction seen clinically. Zimmerman et al.[15] described similar findings in 52 osteoporotic patients treated with either percutaneous pinning and cast immobilization for 6 weeks or Norian SRS augmented pin or screw fixation with immobilization for 3 weeks and pin removal at 4 weeks. At 2 years, the cement group had better DASH scores and less loss of reduction.

Collectively, these studies have yielded important findings that may be used to guide clinical management. When used alone, calcium phosphate bone cement is likely inadequate for most fracture types. However, there may be circumstances where the early return of motion and avoidance of all hardware may outweigh the potential consequences of poorer long-term radiologic findings. Elderly patients who require early mobilization to perform required activities of daily living and do not want to risk the potential complications of K wires are one such population. K wires may be placed, if desired, to add support without prolonging immobilization, with the knowledge that the likelihood of reduction maintenance in the long-term will be higher.

Most severe fracture types today however, are treated with open reduction and internal fixation using various plating methods. It is probable that the more severely comminuted and unstable fractures, will benefit from the adjunctive use of bone cement. Though outcome studies like the ones described above for K-wire fixation have not been performed, several case studies and techniques have been described in the literature.

Technique

The techniques and potential benefits described in this section are based on our own experience and those of other surgeons who have contributed to the literature [16-18]. With the most complex fracture types, open reduction with plate fixation with or without external fixation or K-wire fixation may still be inadequate. When cancellous bone is crushed leaving a void, or articular fragments are small or missing, calcium phosphate cement can be a helpful adjunct.

Surgery is performed under general or block anesthesia. The fracture is approached first via a standard volar approach through the bed of the flexor carpi radialis tendon. The extent of comminution is assessed and the fracture fragments are reduced as well as possible. This often necessitates a separate dorsal incision that allows direct visualization of the joint surface and better control of the dorsal medial intraarticular fragments. K-wires may be used to temporarily maintain reduction before plate application. At this point, bone cement could potentially be used to assist with holding the reduction. It would require the consistency of putty, yet not cure so quickly or become so hard that it cannot be removed. We have not found a cement that meets these requirements and therefore apply our plate before cement introduction in most cases. Fragment and plate position is confirmed by fluoroscopy. If the dorsal cortex is not highly comminuted and appears stable, no additional hardware is used. The calcium phosphate cement is then used to fill all voids.

We have used HydroSet (Stryker, Kalamazoo, MI, USA). While a low viscosity cement is imperative for percutaneous application, this property is less important when using an open technique. The advantage of a syringe-loaded cement is that it can completely fill the metaphyseal void and seal any space between the plated fragments. Our experience with HydroSet is that there is a quick setting time and ability to set in a wet field. However, when there is no clearly defined cavity (often the case with severely comminuted distal radius fractures) cement is prone to extrusion. Extruded cement may cause synovitis, tendonitis, or local pain and should be removed if possible. We have also found that manipulating it while setting, causes the material to become chalky and brittle.

In addition to being used as a void filler, the cement theoretically can be used to secure cortical and articular fragments too small to hold a screw or K-wire. Though not ideal, in certain cases when portions of the articular surface are destroyed or missing, calcium phosphate cement can be used to replace the missing articular surface. In one case, HydroSet was used to reconstruct 80% of an articular surface.

Though the cement is marketed as being able to hold screws, we have not found this to be possible.

Case Series

Methods

All consecutive severely comminuted distal radius fractures treated by the senior author in our institution over a period of 9 months using standard surgical technique and rigid fixation were reviewed. Patient mean age was 50.7. There were 33 distal radius fractures treated surgically. HydroSet bone cement was used in 14 fractures in 14 patients. The indications for using the cement were severe comminution and bone loss and the surgeon's judgment of technical inability to obtain rigid fixation due to insufficient bone.

Results

In 9 out of the 13 cases a dorsal approach was used in addition to a volar. In all cases, a 2.4 mm stainless steel volar locking plate (Synthes) was used. Severe dorsal comminution with loss of articular surface and articular support was present in 9 cases. In all of these, calcium phosphate bone cement was used to reconstruct the dorsal articular surface. All patients but one went on to bony healing without collapse on X-rays at 6 weeks follow-up. Average flexion extension arc at 5 months was 120 degrees (50-180). The patients with the most severe intra-articular involvement had the lower range of motion scores. Radiographs following surgery were remarkable for bone graft in the soft tissues especially when the graft had been used to reconstruct the dorsal bone. Four patients required further surgery. All of these patients had their hardware removed. The patient who demonstrated collapse had a partial nonunion (the radial styloid fragment healed to the shaft but a large medial articular fragment was not united). Since the fragments were now two large bony fragments, plating was straightforward and no further grafting was needed. In all of the patients, it seemed that the bone cement had been replaced by bone except in the areas where the graft had extruded into the soft tissues. In these areas, the fragments of bone cement were removed at the time of hardware removal.

Discussion

Bone cements are a useful adjunct in the management of difficult distal radius fractures. Though surgeons have employed cements for fractures of varying severity, their greatest utility is likely in highly comminuted, intra-articular fractures. In this setting, bone cement may fill metaphyseal void, provide fracture stabilization during fixation, resurface missing articular surface, secure small fracture fragments, allow for less invasive fixation techniques, avoid the need for autologous bone graft, and overall, make the operation technically easier.

Currently, calcium phosphate/sulfate bone cements are the favored cement for use in distal radius fractures. There are many available formulations that are biocompatibile, osteoconductive, have varying viscosity and consistency, and set quickly with an isothermic reaction. Drawbacks include limited resistance to forces other than axial loading, extrusion during injection, inability to manipulate significantly during hardening, and fracture with screw placement.

In our case series, HydroSet bone cement was a useful adjunct to internal fixation in a population of patients with highly comminuted, intra-articular fractures. The cement allowed for better retention of reduction and allowed for less invasive fixation techniques as our experience with the technique matured. Bony healing with maintenance of radial height was achieved in all but one patient. During revision surgeries the cement was noted to be replaced by bone. We have found this cement to be a useful adjunct to plate fixation techniques and offer the following as key points:

1. In most cases, bone cement should not be used alone. Appropriate hardware may be selected according to the situation and surgeon preference.
2. Cement should not be manipulated too much while it hardens as it may compromise its integrity.
3. Screw insertion into cement should be avoided as it may result in cement fracture.
4. Cement may be used to fill gaps between fragments, hold fragments too small to support hardware, and resurface the articular surface.
5. Cement that has extruded into soft tissue or the joint space should be removed if possible. Cement in soft tissue has not resulted in ectopic bone formation in our experience.
6. Use of bone cement should allow for less invasive fixation techniques and earlier motion

Though the properties of these cements are not ideal and their role in distal radius fracture management is not well established, familiarity with the products can prove useful when dealing with challenging fractures.

References

[1] McQueen, MM; MacLaren, A. J. Chalmers, The value of remanipulating Colles' fractures. *J Bone Joint Surg Br.*, 1986, 68(2), p. 232-3.

[2] Handoll, HH; Madhok, R. Surgical interventions for treating distal radial fractures in adults. *Cochrane Database Syst Rev.*, 2003, (3), p. CD003209.

[3] Arora, J; Malik, AC. External fixation in comminuted, displaced intra-articular fractures of the distal radius: is it sufficient? *Arch Orthop Trauma Surg.*, 2005, 125(8), p. 536-40.

[4] Weber, SC; Szabo, RM. Severely comminuted distal radial fracture as an unsolved problem: complications associated with external fixation and pins and plaster techniques. *J Hand Surg* [Am], 1986, 11(2), p. 157-65.

[5] Bartucci, EJ; et al, The effect of adjunctive methylmethacrylate on failures of fixation and function in patients with intertrochanteric fractures and osteoporosis. *J Bone Joint Surg Am*, 1985, 67(7), p. 1094-107.

[6] Schatzker, J; Ha'eri, GB; Chapman, M. Methylmethacrylate as an adjunct in the internal fixation of intertrochanteric fractures of the femur. *J Trauma*, 1978, 18(10), p. 732-5.

[7] Schmalholz, A. Bone cement for redislocated Colles' fracture. A prospective comparison with closed treatment. *Acta Orthop Scand*, 1989, 60(2), p. 212-7.

[8] Schmalholz, A. External skeletal fixation versus cement fixation in the treatment of redislocated Colles' fracture. *Clin Orthop Relat Res*., 1990, (254), p. 236-41.

[9] Urban, RM; et al. Increased bone formation using calcium sulfate-calcium phosphate composite graft. *Clin Orthop Relat Res*., 2007, 459, p. 110-7.

[10] Yetkinler, DN; et al. Biomechanical evaluation of fixation of intra-articular fractures of the distal part of the radius in cadavera: Kirschner wires compared with calcium-phosphate bone cement. *J Bone Joint Surg Am*, 1999, 81(3), p. 391-9.

[11] Higgins, TF; Dodds, SD; Wolfe, SW. A biomechanical analysis of fixation of intra-articular distal radial fractures with calcium-phosphate bone cement. *J Bone Joint Surg Am*, 2002, 84-A(9), p. 1579-86.

[12] Sanchez-Sotelo, J; Munuera, L. Madero, R. Treatment of fractures of the distal radius with a remodellable bone cement: a prospective, randomised study using Norian SRS. *J Bone Joint Surg Br*, 2000, 82(6), p. 856-63.

[13] Kopylov, P; et al, *Norian SRS versus external fixation in redisplaced distal radial fractures. A randomized study in 40 patients. Acta Orthop Scand*, 1999, 70(1), p. 1-5.

[14] Jeyam, M; et al, *Controlled trial of distal radial fractures treated with a resorbable bone mineral substitute. J Hand Surg* [Br], 2002. 27(2), p. 146-9.

[15] Zimmermann, R; et al, Injectable calcium phosphate bone cement Norian SRS for the treatment of intra-articular compression fractures of the distal radius in osteoporotic women. *Arch Orthop Trauma Surg*., 2003, 123(1), p. 22-7.

[16] Huber, FX; et al. Open reduction and palmar plate-osteosynthesis in combination with a nanocrystalline hydroxyapatite spacer in the treatment of comminuted fractures of the distal radius. *J Hand Surg* [Br], 2006. 31(3), p. 298-303.

[17] Kamano, M; et al. Palmar plating system for Colles' fractures--a preliminary report. *J Hand Surg* [Am], 2005, 30(4), p. 750-5.

[18] Gangopadhyay, S; Ravi, K; Packer, G. Dorsal plating of unstable distal radius fractures using a bio-absorbable plating system and bone substitute. *J Hand Surg* [Br], 2006, 31(1), p. 93-100.

In: Hand Surgery: Preoperative Expectations...
Editor: Robert H. Beckingsworth
ISBN: 978-1-60876-280-4

Chapter 8

Intramedullary Fixation of Distal Radius Fractures

Neil R. Macintyre[1] ***and Asif M. Ilyas***[2*]
[1]Department of Orthopaedic Surgery Temple University Hospital, Philadelphia, PA, USA
[2]Temple Hand Center Assistant Professor, Department of Orthopaedic Surgery, Temple University Hospital, Philadelphia, PA, USA

Abstract

The goal of internal fixation of the distal radius fracture is restoration of the disrupted anatomy and early return to function while minimizing soft tissue trauma and prolonged immobilization. This has been achieved with standard plating techniques, particularly volar locked-plates. More recently, intramedullary fixation has experienced increased interest as an alternate option for distal radius fracture fixation. Intramedullary fixation permits limited soft tissue dissection and insertion of a low profile that acts as an internal splint. The use of intramedullary fixation for displaced distal radius fractures utilizes the accepted principles of stable fracture fixation and early motion but also provides the additional benefits of load-sharing and decreased soft tissue irritation. Purported benefits include a familiar fracture fixation technique, less soft tissue irritation, and locked fixed-angle technology.

Thorough understanding of the radial and dorsal approaches to the distal radius is a prerequisite. Surgical technique involves (1) fracture reduction, (2) nail insertion, and (3) locking screw placement. Important aspects of intramedullary fixation of distal radius fractures include proper fracture selection, good fracture reduction, protection of sensory nerves, and avoidance of inadvertent intra-articular screw placement. Fractures indicated for intramedullary fixation include predominantly displaced extra-articular or simple intra-articular distal radius fractures.

* Corresponding Author: ASIF ILYAS, MD TUH – Department of Orthopaedic Surgery 6th Floor Outpt Bldg – Zone B 3401 N. Broad Street Philadelphia, PA 19140; Phone: 215-694-4850; Email: asif.ilyas@tuhs.temple.edu

Background

The earliest description of the wrist injury that is known today as a distal radius fracture was provided by Pouteau and Colles prior to the age of x-rays. Colles in particular was able to accurately describe the nature and common dorsal alignment of the wrist following a distal radius fracture but he also assumed "that the limb will at some remote period again enjoy perfect freedom in all of its motions and be completely exempt from pain."[1] In contrast, today we recognize that distal radius fractures are complex injuries that can benefit from a myriad of treatment options.

Operative treatment options include percutaneous pinning, external fixation, and open reduction internal fixation. The goal of internal fixation of the distal radius fracture is restoration of the disrupted anatomy and early return to function while minimizing soft tissue trauma and prolonged immobilization. Recently, intramedullary fixation has experienced increased interest as an alternate option for distal radius fracture fixation. (Figure 1) Intramedullary fixation permits limited soft tissue dissection and insertion of a low profile implant that acts as an internal splint. The use of intramedullary fixation for displaced distal radius fractures utilizes the accepted principles of stable fracture fixation and early motion but also provides the additional benefits of load-sharing and decreased soft tissue irritation. Purported benefits include a familiar fracture fixation technique, less soft tissue irritation, and fixed-angle locking technology.

Intramedullary Nailing

Intramedullary nailing first gained popularity in the 1940's through the work of Dr. Kuntscher. Over the past 60 years techniques and implants have evolved that affords intramedullary fixation of nearly every long bone in the body. Intramedullary fixation provides multiple advantages in the management of fractures including reliable bone healing, minimal disruption to periosteal blood supply, less soft tissue irritation, early weight-bearing, and earlier range of motion.

Specific to the distal radius, intramedullary fixation similarly provides limited soft tissue disruption with a zero profile implant in an area of the wrist otherwise intimately enveloped by closely approximated soft tissue. Also, intramedullary fixation provides the important principles of stable fracture fixation and reliable healing. Cumulatively, these design advantages facilitates initiation of early hand and wrist motion, improved tendon gliding, decreased swelling, and avoidance of disuse osteopenia..

Surgical Indications

Utilizing the AO Classification, the primary indication for use of intramedullary fixation for distal radius fractures are displaced extra-articular AO Type A fractures. [2] In addition, intramedullary fixation can also be used for predominantly extra-articular fractures with only simple intra-articular extension, or AO Type C1 fractures. (Figure 2)

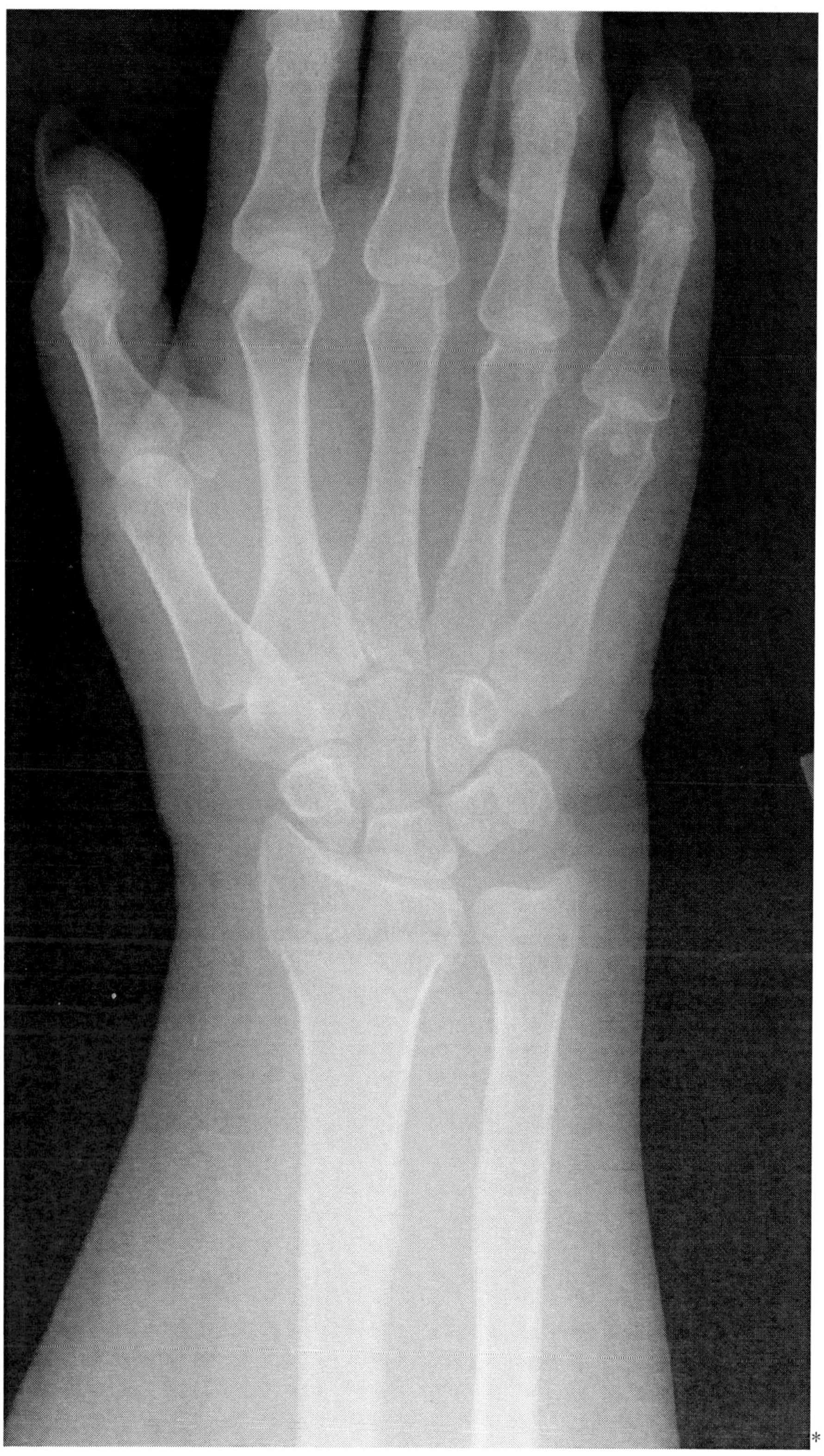

Figure 1. Implant attached to insertion jig ex vivo.

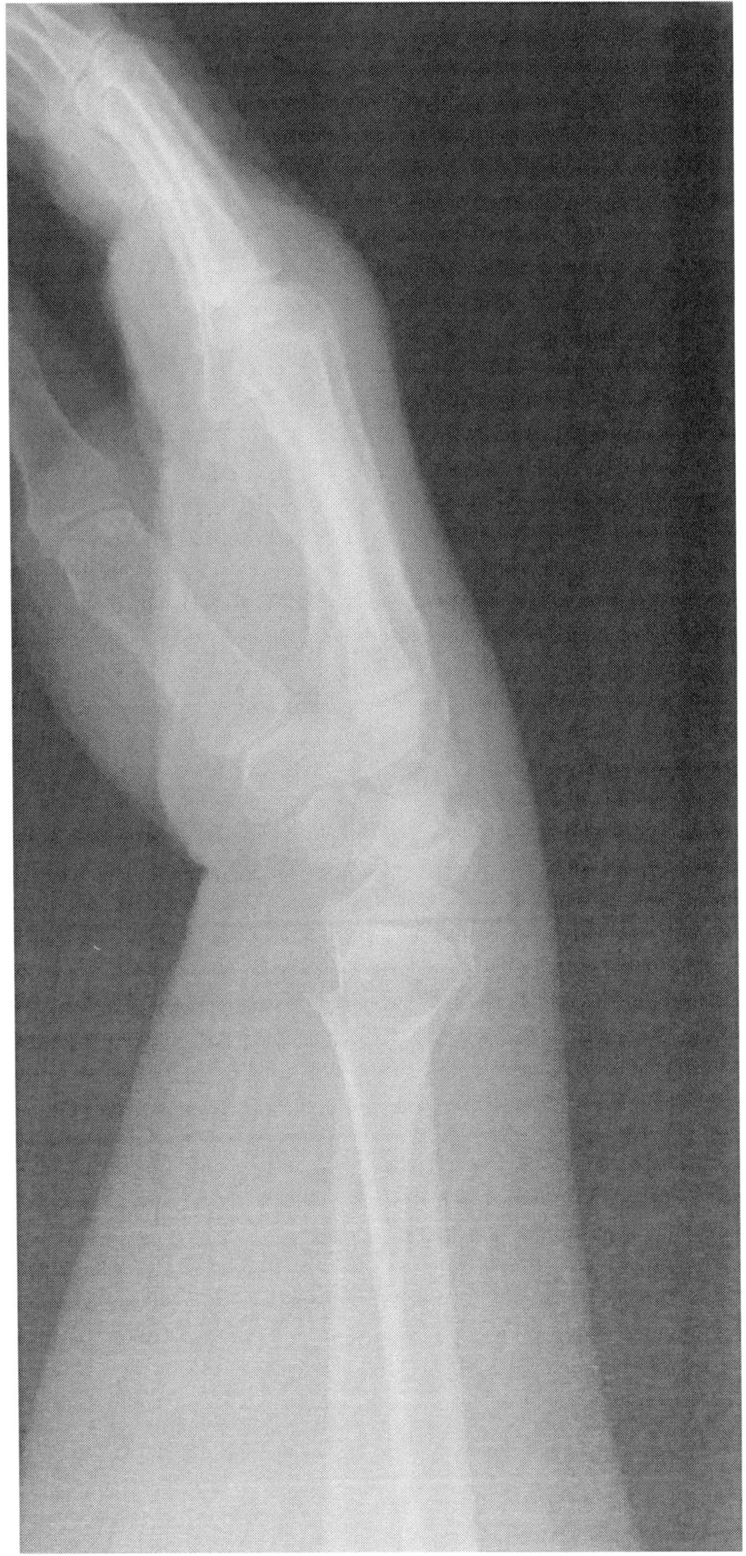

Figure 2. Predominantly extra-articular distal radius fracture indicated for intramedullary fixation.

Marginal rim or shear fracture configurations (ie, the volar or dorsal Barton's fractures and other AO Type B patterns), and fractures with multiple and/or significantly displaced intra-articular fragments (AO Type C2 and C3) are contraindicated due to the intramedullary device's limitations in direct articular fracture reduction and internal fixation.

Additional contraindications include pediatric fractures with open physes, open fractures, and the presence of active local infection or inadequate wound coverage.

Surgical Technique

Intramedullary fixation of the distal radius utilizes both a limited radial and dorsal approach to the wrist. (Figure 3) The radial approach is utilized for nail insertion and distal locking screw placement. The dorsal approach is utilized for placement of the nail's proximal inter-locking screws as well as for limited open fracture reduction, if necessary.

All surgeries should be performed with general or regional anesthesia, tourniquet hemostasis, and fluoroscopic assistance. The first step involves closed reduction of the fracture under fluoroscopy. Once the fracture is adequately reduced with restoration of normal distal radius parameters percutaneously pin the fracture along the dorsal ulnar column of the distal radius. (Figure 4) Placement of the pin will facilitate maintenance of fracture reduction during the remaining procedure.

Often closed means for fracture reduction prove inadequate, particularly if the fracture is shingled along the volar cortex. In these circumstances a limited dorsal incision can be made to facilitate direct open reduction of the fracture. This same dorsal incision can later be used for placement of the proximal inter-locking screws.

Once the fracture is adequately reduced and pinned, place a 2-3 cm incision along the distal radial column of the radius. Branches of the superficial radial sensory nerve should be actively identified and diligently protected throughout the remaining procedure. Identify the interval between the first and second dorsal compartments in a sub-periosteal fashion. The compartments themselves do not need to be opened.

Create an opening in the radial aspect of the distal radius with a guidewire and reamer and direct an awl into the distal radius' intramedullary canal. (FIGURE 5) The awl should be allowed to bluntly find the intramedullary canal of the radius. After the awl identifies the path, sequentially broach the canal across the fracture. Broach the radius until a good proximal fill of the radius is achieved. A tight fit is not necessary. After broaching, the nail is sized and trialed. Use fluoroscopic guidance regularly to guide placement of the implants and to avoid inadvertent injury to the articular surfaces or loss of fracture reduction.

The nail and insertion jig are assembled on the backtable. (FIGURE 1) Insert the nail so that the subchondral locking screws will be sufficiently below the distal radius articular surface. Once confirmed, place the divergent fixed-angle locking subchondral screws through the insertion jig. These screws turn the nail into a fixed-angle device within the distal fracture fragment. In addition to avoiding screw penetration of the articular surface, diligent protection of the branches of the radial sensory nerve again must be maintained.

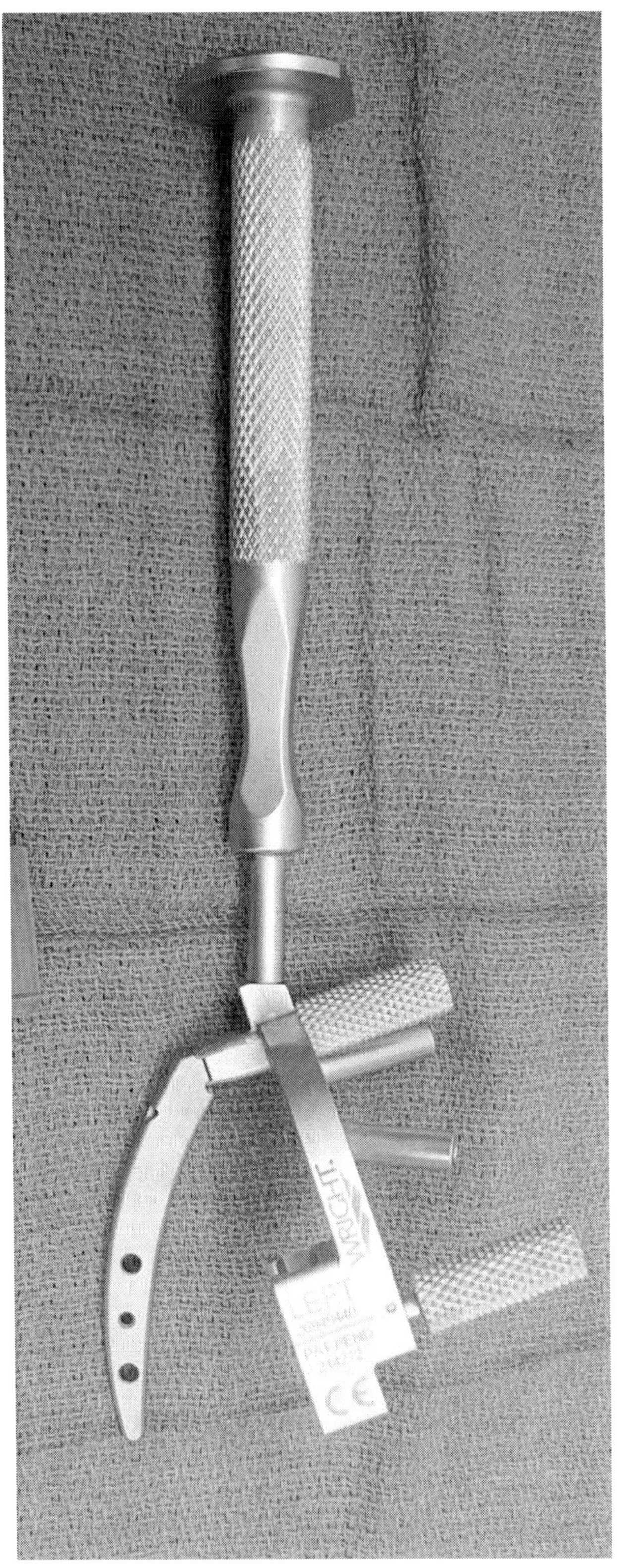

Figure 3. Markings for the radial and dorsal approaches to the distal radius.

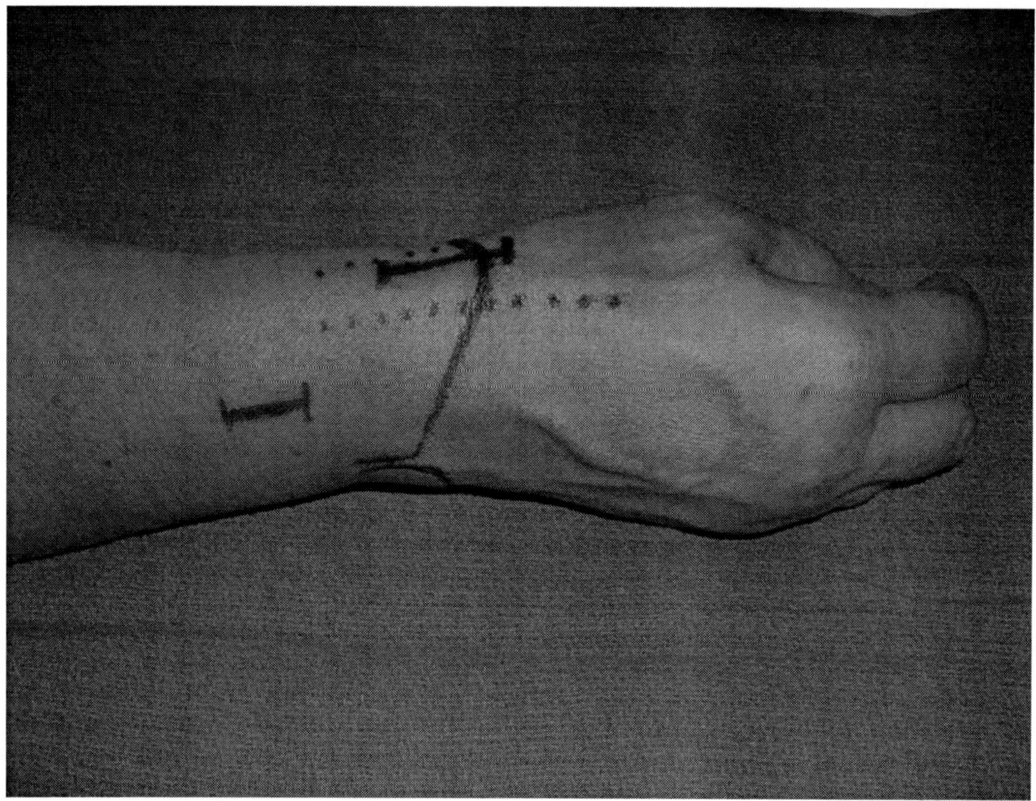

Figure 4. Closed reduction and pinning of the fracture.

Following creation of a fixed-angle device distally, the nail can be inter-locked proximally and final position of the nail and fracture fixed. Proximal nail fixation is achieved with dorsal placement of bicortical screws. A 2 cm incision is placed approximately 1 cm proximal to Lister's tubercle and blunt dissection is used down to the dorsal surface of the radius. Using the aiming guide on the insertion jig place the proximal inter-locking screws through the dorsal cortex. The screws should be bicortical for adequate fixation.

Final images should confirm reduction and fixation of the fracture. (FIGURE 6) Close the skin incisions with 4-0 nylon sutures. After dressing the wound, apply a volar plaster splint with the metacarpophalangeal joints and fingers free. Within 2 weeks after surgery, the splint and sutures should be removed and motion initiated under the supervision of a therapist.

Surgical Pearls & Pitfalls

Successful use of intramedullary fixation of distal radius fractures begins with proper fracture selection. The intramedullary nail should be limited to primarily extra-articular fractures. Distal radius fractures with marginal rim, multiple or displaced intra-articular fractures must be avoided.

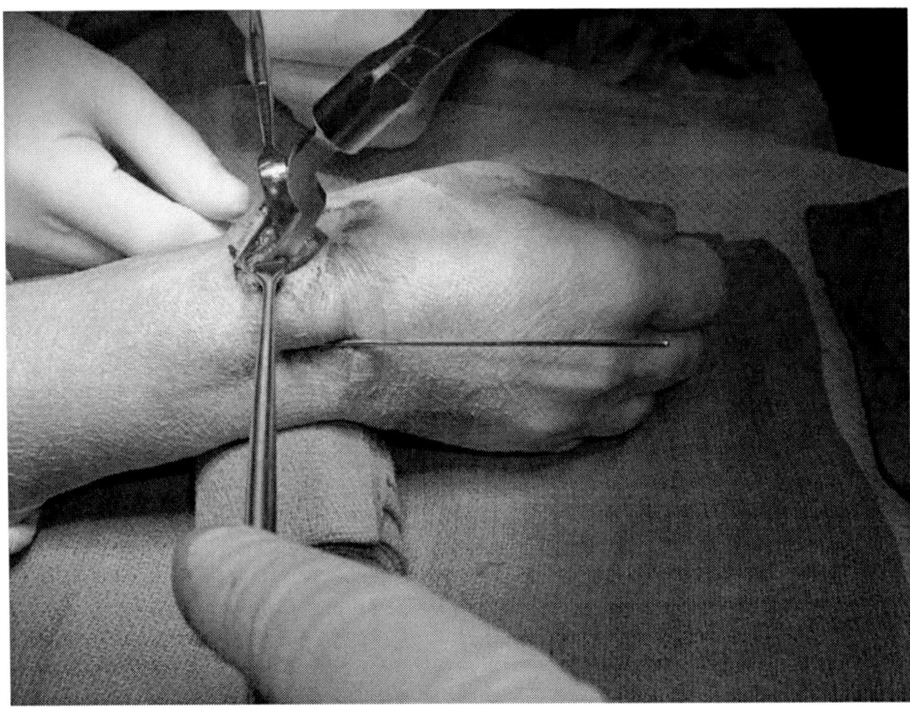

Figure 5. Insertion of the awl into the reduced distal radius fracture through the radial styloid between the first and second dorsal compartments.

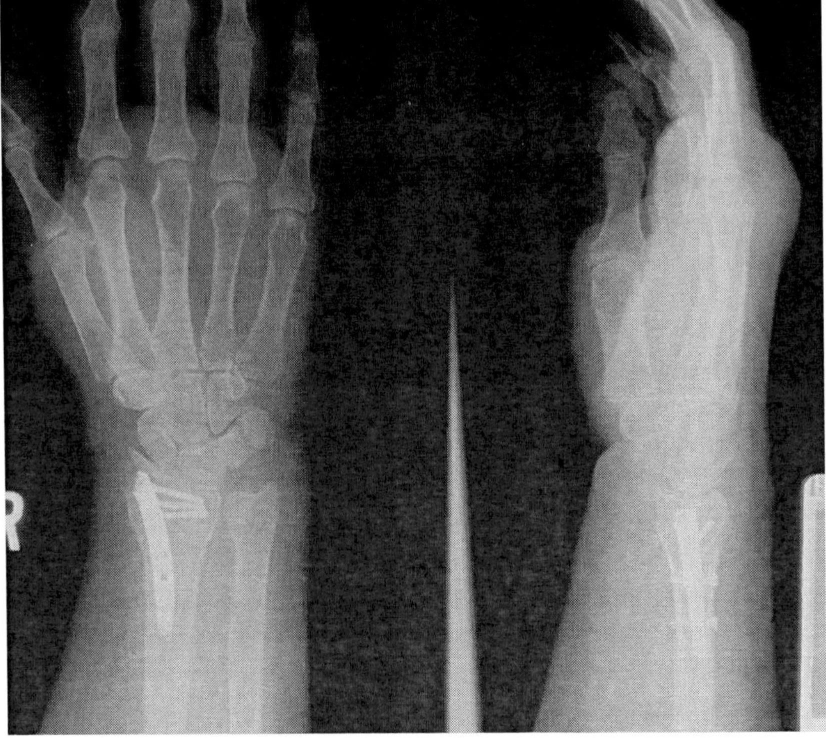

Figure 6. Final images with implant in place.

Good fracture reduction must be achieved prior to reaming and nail insertion. The intramedullary nail once inserted does not facilitate much additional fracture reduction.

The superficial radial sensory nerve is always present in the field of the radial incision and is highly susceptible to direct and indirect injury. All branches must be identified and thoughtfully protected at all times.

The risk of inadvertent articular screw penetration is high and is best avoided by using imaging routinely during screw placement. In particular, the distal radioulnar joint is most susceptible and requires close radiographic evaluation.

After Surgery, Early Wrist Mobilization Should be Initiated

Outcomes and Discussion

There are currently no level I studies at this time evaluating the use of an intramedullary implant in the treatment of distal radius fractures. However, several level IV studies representing case series are available and show early promise. [3-6]

Originally Tan et al described the technique of distal radius intramedullary fixation with the MICRONAIL (Wright Medical, Arlington) and noted that 15 patients treated with this implant showed promising clinical and radiographic results.[3] It should be noted that 3 of 15 patients developed transient radial sensory nerve neuritis which resolved by three months. No further objective measurements were reported.

In follow up to this series, Brooks et al reported on an unpublished series of 23 patients with distal radius fractures treated with the MICRONAIL.[4,5] The series consisted of unstable distal radius fractures consisting of AO Type A2, A3, B3, C1, and C2. At six month follow-up the average flexion was 58 degrees and extension was 73 degrees, ulnar deviation 28 degrees, radial deviation of 22 degrees, supination of 78 degrees, and pronation of 87 degrees. Grip strength measured 80% of the contralateral limb. All but three patients maintained fracture reduction to final follow-up, except two C2 cases and one B3 case. Again transient radial sensory nerve neuritis was noted in three patints which resolved within 2 months. The average DASH score was an 8.0. No cases of infection, complex regional pain syndrome, hardware failure, of soft tissue irritation occurred.

Ilyas & Thoder followed 10 patients over a 21 month period who were treated with the same intramedullary implant for AO type A and C1 fractures.[6] At final follow-up they identified an average volar tilt of 2.2 degrees of dorsal angulation, radial inclination of 24.1 degreees, radial height of 12.1 mm, radial inclination of 24.1 degrees, and ulnar variance of -0.6 mm. All but two cases maintained post operative reduction. Both cases represented A3 fractures and resulted in a greater than 5 degrees loss of volar tilt. Pronation was 85 degrees while supination was 82 degrees. Wrist flexion was noted to be 67 degrees and wrist extension at 71 degrees. Grip strength was noted to be 91% of the contralateral limb. The average DASH score was 8.1 with 8 excellent, 1 good, and 1 poor. Complications included 2 cases of transient superficial radial sensory neuritis and 3 cases of DRUJ screw penetration. No cases of infection, tendon injury, or hardware failure were reported.

Conclusion

In summary, the use of intramedullary fixation for displaced distal radius fractures utilizes the accepted principles of stable fracture fixation and early motion but also provides the additional benefits of load-sharing and decreased soft tissue irritation. If used for appropriately indicated patients, intramedullary fixation can provide excellent results.

References

[1] Colles, A. On the fracture of the carpal extremity of the radius. *Edinb Med Surg J.* 1814, 10, 181.

[2] Muller, ME; Nazarian, S; Koch, P; Schatzker, J. The comprehensive classification of fractures of long bones. *Berlin:Springer-Verlag*, 1990, 106-15.

[3] Tan, V, Capo, J, Warburton, M. Distal Radius Fracture Fixation with and Intramedullary Nail. *Tech Hand Up Extrem Surg*, 2005, 9, 195-201

[4] Tan, V; Capo, JT; Warburton, M. Minimally invasive Distal Radius Fracture Fixation with an Intramedullary Nail. Annual Meeting of the American Society for Surgery of the Hand (ASSH), 2005, San Antonio, TX

[5] Brooks, KR; Capo, JT; Warburton, M; Tan, V. Internal Fixation of Distal Radius Fractures with Novel Intramedullary Implants. *Clinical Orthopaedics and Related Research*, 2006, 445, 42-50

[6] Ilyas, AM; Thoder, JJ. Intramedullary Fixation of Displaced Distal Radius Fractures: A Preliminary Report. *J Hand Surgery*, 2008, 33A, 1706-1715

In: Hand Surgery: Preoperative Expectations...
Editor: Robert H. Beckingsworth

ISBN: 978-1-60876-280-4

Chapter 9

Degradable Polymers in Hand Surgery*

***Abigail R. Hamilton*[1], *Chaitanya S. Mudgal*[†1,2] *and Jesse B. Jupiter*[3]**

[1] Harvard Combined Orthopaedic Surgery Residency Program
Massachusetts General Hospital, 55 Fruit Street, Boston, MA 02114,USA

[2] Massachusetts General Hospital, Instructor, Orthopaedic Surgery
Harvard Medical School, Yawkey Center, Suite 2100
55 Fruit Street, Boston, MA 02114, USA

[3] Massachusetts General Hospital, Hansjorg Wyss / AO Professor of Orthopaedic Surgery, Harvard Medical School, Yawkey Center, Suite 2100
55 Fruit Street, Boston, MA 02114, USA

Abstract

Implants used in the hand and wrist have to satisfy certain criteria. They should be small, biomechanically strong enough to withstand loading in the hand and wrist and should have a low profile. In addition to these features, it is extremely useful, if they are inert enough to avoid causing local soft tissue or bony reaction and therefore do not require additional procedures for removal. Bioabsorbable implants fulfill all these criteria, and although their use in the hand and wrist is still in its infancy, early data suggest that the rates of success and complications associated with their use, are comparable to that associated with their metal counterparts. As costs associated with their

---

* A version of this chapter was also published in Degradable Polymers for Skeletal Implants, edited by Paul. I. J. M. Wuisman and Theo H. Smit published by Nova Science Publishers, Inc. It was submitted for appropriate modifications in an effort to encourage wider dissemination of research.

† Address for Correspondence:Chaitanya S. Mudgal, MD, MS(Orth.), M.Ch(Orth.)Orthopaedic Hand Service,Massachusetts General Hospital,Instructor, Orthopaedic Surgery,Harvard Medical School,Yawkey Center, Suite 2100,55 Fruit Street,Boston, MA 02114.,Telephone: 617 643 3945,Fax : 617 724 8532,Email : cmudgal@partners.org.

production and use reduce, and more data regarding their efficacy become available, it appears that universal acceptance will follow.

Introduction

Over the past few decades, there has been a shift in the treatment of hand fractures from non-operative immobilization techniques to a more surgically oriented approach. An important component of this shift has been the production of mini- and micro-plating systems and implantation devices specific to the complex needs of the hand. The interplay of intricate ligamentous, capsular and tendinous structures of the hand make development of these implants challenging since implant strength needs to be balanced with a low profile and small size.

The first mini and micro-plating systems were initially developed for use in craniomaxillofacial surgery and were then transferred to use in surgical procedures on the hand. The use of bio-absorbable compounds has followed this same progression with the most extensive use documented and studied within the field of craniomaxillofacial surgery. Long-term follow-up of over ten years of use is available mainly within craniomaxillofacial literature [5] and remains largely unavailable within hand surgery due to its relatively new implementation. The clinical results available are mainly composed of small cohorts of case series or retrospective reviews. Large cohorts of patients have been reviewed retrospectively but include fractures from all anatomic areas and are not specific to hand surgery [8, 33].

Suture materials were the first bio-absorbable devices used within surgery but since the late 1980s the use of other bio-absorbable devices including pins, rods, suture anchors, plates and screws in procedures specific to the hand has been increasing. Interest in bio-absorbable compounds within hand surgery arises from its potential ability to have strength to maintain anatomic reduction during osseous healing and then degrade when no longer required therefore eliminating the potential need for future hardware removal. Another potential benefit is the radiolucency of bio-absorbable implants allowing for ease in radiographic follow-up in the assessment of osseous healing. The implants also do not interfere with computed tomography (CT) or magnetic resonance (MR) imaging causing the scatter effect typically seen with metallic implants. Rigid metallic devices are known to be associated with osteopenia deep to the plate that may lead to re-fracture; this osteopenia and its effects may also be decreased by the less rigid fixation of bio-absorbable devices.

The new technology is not without its own complications, most notably local irritation of soft tissues from foreign body reactions resulting in local swelling, effusions and sinus tract formation [8, 39]. Another limitation to widespread use is the cost and restricted availability of implants compared with metallic implants. Due to the decreased strength of bioabsorbable implants, they are not designed to be either self-drilling or self-tapping [39]. Previous experience and practice is strongly recommended in order to achieve the best clinical outcomes, as their use may be more technically demanding [39]. Accurate fracture reduction is essential as interfragmentary compression with miniscrews is not possible and bioabsorbable pins are less forgiving and harder to remove than Kirschner wires requiring re-drilling in some cases.

The proper rationale must be applied in each surgical case to determine if a bio-absorbable implant may be of benefit to a patient. However, with further materials science research, industry production of implants as well as ongoing basic science and clinical research, bio-absorbable implants may offer new possibilities in the armamentarium of treatment options for hand surgeons.

Bio-Absorbable Compounds

As a full review of bio-absorbable compounds is available in Chapter X, this will be a brief overview of bio-absorbable compounds available for use in surgery specific to the hand. Of the numerous bio-absorbable polymers available for medical use, in-depth study of osteofixation devices has focused on high molecular weight polyhydroxyacids formed by ring-opening polymerization of cyclic diesters, polyglycolide [PGA], polylactide [PLA] and their copolymers. PLA is the cyclic dimer of lactic acid existing as two optical isomers, D and L. PLA is seen in implants as polylevolactic acid (PLLA) or various ratios of copolymers of polylevo- and polydextrolactic acid (P(L/DL)LA). The strength characteristics of these polymers have been further enhanced with the development of self-reinforcing (SR-devices). These compounds have been used in a multitude of procedures in surgical treatment of hand disorders given their biocompatibility, inherent mechanical properties and the ability to adjust degradation rates by varying their composition.

***Biodegradation*:** Degradation of bio-absorbable polymers occurs mainly via hydrolysis. However, in vivo testing has also implicated enzymatic degradation processes to a lesser extent [43]. In vivo, PLA and PGA are degraded to lactic acid and glycine which produce carbon dioxide and water via the citric acid cycle with byproducts excreted mainly via respiration. The acidic byproducts produced in the initial stages (lactic acid and glycine) further act to catalyze the degradation over time as well as to create an acidic environment relative to surrounding tissues, an occurrence which has been theorized to produce an environment adverse to bacterial ingrowth [2, 5]. Final elimination of polymeric debris is thought to be a function of macrophages and giant cells.

Degradation rates vary, with PLLA having the longest degradation time due to the crystallinity and hydrophobicity of the compound from methyl groups, while PGA degrades faster due to the hydrophilic nature of the compound. As with any compound, the chemical make-up, the porosity, surface to volume ratio and sterilization method affect degradation time. Specific to the bio-absorbable polymers used are the size of the polymer, geometric isomerization, monomer concentration and crystallinity. Work by Vasenius et al. shows that in vivo degradation is faster than in vitro and is also increased based on host factors such as vascularity of surrounding tissues, mechanical stress and implantation site [43]. In this study, degradation was noted to be faster in well vascularized cancellous bone than in subcutaneous tissue. Cellular enzymes have been described to enhance degradation of polymers and a vascular environment rich in cellular elements may explain the faster rate of degradation in bone [42]. Loss of strength occurs prior to macroscopically detectable degradation of implants [33]. Clinically, the absorption time for SR-PGA is 6-12 months [34]. Pure PLLA make take 5 years or more to fully degrade and P(L/DL)LA implants between 2-3 years [6].

Mechanical properties: A multitude of factors affect the mechanical properties of bio-absorbable implants. The most important being their biochemical structure and composition, the technique used to produce the implant, and sterilization technique.

The homopolymer of the L isomer of PLA (PLLA) is a semicrystalline polymer which exhibits high tensile strength and low elongation. This results in a high modulus that makes them more suitable for load-bearing applications required in orthopedic fixation and sutures. These polymers exhibit a glass-transition temperature. Above this temperature the material is soft and malleable. In non-SR devices, heating above this transition temperature is required for plate molding. PLLA is about 37% crystalline with a glass-transition temperature of 60—65°C. P(L/DL)LA is an amorphous polymer exhibiting a random distribution of both isomeric forms of lactic acid, and accordingly is unable to arrange into an organized crystalline structure. This effectively decreases the modulus as the percentage of D-isomer presence increases. PGA is an amorphous material with a glass-transition temperature of approximately 36°C.

Clinical studies reveal that in vivo, strength of SR-PLLA implants decreases overtime and becomes equivalent to the strength of cancellous bone in 36 weeks [24]. Complete mechanical strength of SR-P(L/DL)LA 70/30 occurs in approximately four months.

Available Implant Devices

Implant production using bio-absorbable polymers is performed via multiple techniques. Production via melt-extrusion, injection molding and compression molding have all been reported in early production. Implants produced via these techniques are usually brittle and flexible and are unsuitable for areas of high stress. In 1992 Tormala introduced self-reinforcing as a manufacturing technique revolutionizing the use of bio-absorbable implants in osteosynthesis. This involves formation of a composite polymer structure with reinforcing units of the same chemical structure laid in parallel with a binding matrix. This technique produces high-strength implants that can be molded at room temperature with routine plate bending techniques as opposed to non-reinforced plates that require heating above their glass transition temperature prior to contouring [37, 39]. This self-reinforcing technique also allows for sterilization with γ-irradiation without significant loss of strength of the implant.

Clinical Applications

Distal Radius

In recent history there has been a large influx of new implant designs available commercially for the treatment of distal radius fractures. While the role of internal fixation has increased in the treatment of unstable fractures with this influx, it is not without its own complications. Flexor and extensor tendon irritation have been reported at a rate of over 10 % [4, 11, 12, 19, 32] and tendon ruptures have also been reported. Recent introduction of a bioabsorbable dorsal distal radius plate offers a potential solution to the need for implant removal because of persistent tendon irritation which has been reported at a rate of 12-23% [11, 12, 19, 32].

Gangopadhyay et. al reported results of treatment of 26 unstable, intraarticular dorsally displaced fractures of the distal radius with a bioabsorbable dorsal distal radius plate (ReUnite) and calcium phosphate (Biobon) bone substitute. The Reunite plate is a copolymer of PLLA and PGA (82%/18%) with a height of 2.5 mm available in small and large sizes. The implant is heated above the glass transition temperature with a portable heat plate to produce malleability for contouring. Five patients lost the reduction achieved at time of surgery, one at 6 weeks and four between 6 and 12 weeks. On re-operation, in the patient who lost reduction at 6 weeks the plate was found to be broken and was revised with a metal plate and iliac crest bone graft. These authors noted severe dorsal comminution in all patients who lost operative reduction and concluded that use of this plating system should not be recommended for fracture fixation, if a metaphyseal gap of greater than 7 mm is noted following open fracture reduction. Other complications included rupture of the long extensor of the thumb and long finger, two cases of extensor tenosynovitis that resolved with 2 weeks of anti-inflammatory medication and splinting and two cases of inflammatory reaction to plate resorption between 8 and 11 weeks. In the cases of the foreign body reactions, one patient was treated with aspiration and one required a return to the operating room for a formal debridement. Both of these patients had an excellent functional result at final review [15].

Further study of bio-absorbable implants in treatment of distal radius fractures will help determine their potential role. Patient perception in the United Kingdom is promising for this research. One hundred consecutive adults with distal radius fractures were interviewed and given detailed information regarding bioabsorbable plating vs. metal plating techniques with 95% reporting that they appreciated the bioabsorbable feature, 91% felt that potential need for removal was the most negative aspect of metal plating techniques and 80% stated they would be willing to participate in a randomized controlled trial to compare the use of the two. The most common concern reported by 29% of patients regarding the bioabsorbable implant was regarding the strength [25].

Wrist Arthrodesis

Wrist arthrodesis is considered the gold-standard of treatment options for painful degenerative joint disease of the wrist. Multiple fixation techniques have been used to effectively stabilize the wrist while fusion occurs, including pins, staples as well as metal plate and screw fixation [18, 27, 31]. Arthrodesis procedures are valuable in both osteoarthritis and rheumatoid disease of the wrist. Rates of fusion throughout the literature reach 96-100% among the various techniques; however complication rates up to 23% have been reported [31]. Due to the relatively common occurrence of secondary procedures for removal of metal pins, plates or screws for migration or discomfort, bio-absorbable implant use in wrist arthrodesis could offer a significant benefit in this area [31].

The most commonly performed surgical technique implementing bio-absorbable implant was initially described by Juutilainen and Patiala in 1995. This technique involves implantation of a SR-PLLA rod (3.2 x 50 mm) in pre-drilled 3.2 mm holes in the distal radius and capitate with the resected ulnar head being utilized as bone graft. Juutilainen and Patiala (1995) described fusion procedures in multiple joints (18 wrist, 18 hand, 6 talocrural, 11 subtalar-calcaneoucuboid-talonavicular joint) in 47 patients with rheumatoid arthritis between 1989 and 1994. They obtained a 100% fusion rate in the wrist and hand with two reported non-unions of the talocrural joint.

Long term results were reviewed by the same group in 21 fusions performed on 18 patients between 1991-1996 with a mean follow-up of 5.4 years with one patient developing a non-union and one patient continued to have severe intermittent pain despite clinical and radiographic evidence of union. In review, complications including infection, median nerve compression, sinus tract formation or aseptic swelling did not occur[46].

Voutilainen et. al (2002) further reported results on 24 wrist arthrodeses in 18 patients with rheumatoid arthritis performed between 1997-2000 using the same technique and obtained fusion in 21 out of 24 cases. One non-union which required re-operation was noted to have rod migration into the medullary canal of the proximal radius and two non-unions did not require further treatment [45]. Satisfactory pain relief was noted in 22 of 24 patients mirroring results reported with metal plates and screws [27]. Patients were followed for an average of 1.7 years and no reports of foreign body reaction were noted. Other than nonunion, there were no other complications.

These initial results are encouraging, and suggest that use of bio-absorbable implants in wrist arthrodesis is as effective at providing stability during fusion as metal implants. They do however, eliminate the morbidity associated with secondary removal of hardware. There is still limited data on fusion in non-rheumatoid patients and long-term follow-up is limited in multiple centers given the new introduction of bio-absorbable implants.

Scaphoid

Treatment of delayed or non-union of scaphoid fractures using various bioabsorbable implants has been reported in literature. Use of quinine dye-coloured SR-PGA pins coated with PDS (2.0 mm diameter) was compared to Herbert Screws (4.0mm diameter) in 34 patients with delayed union or non-union of the scaphoid [28]. Of the 24 patients available to long-term follow-up, (14 in the SR-PGA group and 10 in the Herbert screw group) high complication rates were noted in patients in both groups. Transient sinus formation was reported in 25% of the SR-PGA pin group which was attributed to the color dye and poor vascularity of the scaphoid bone leading to fewer phagocytic cells to absorb the degradation products. Two patients who had Herbert screws placed required removal of the implant due to radiocarpal penetration of the screw. Union rate was reported to be 64% in the SR-PGA group and 60% in the Herbert screw group. However, functional outcome was better in the Herbert screw group.

Yamamuro et. al (1994) reviewed six cases of scaphoid non-union treated with PLLA devices, and noted that union was obtained in all six cases. In their review, there were no noted foreign body reactions [47]. A review of treatment of 12 patients with non-union of the scaphoid with either a SR-PLLA lag screw (6 patients) or two SR-PLLA pins (6 patients), reported a 100% union rate with average time to union of 4.5 months [1]. Four patients had clear drainage from the wound post-operatively that resolved without intervention. These authors noted increased cost to be the major drawback of use of bioabsorbable implants in the treatment of scaphoid nonunion.

Kujala et al. (2004) reported results using non-cannulated 2.0-2.7mm SR-PLLA 70/30 screws in the treatment of 6 patients with scaphoid fractures (3 patients) and non-unions (3 patients). Union was obtained in 5 of 6 patients with one persistent non-union. The authors concluded that bioabsorbable SR-PLLA screws might offer a viable alternative in the treatment of scaphoid non-unions and that the development of cannulated screws over a radio-opaque guide wire may allow more accurate intra-operative positioning of these screws which are radiolucent [21].

Carpus

Trapeziometacarpal (TMC) arthritis: Symptomatic arthritis of the TMC joint often requires surgical intervention. There are a variety of procedures performed including but not limited to ligament reconstruction, osteotomy of the first metacarpal, silicone elastomer arthroplasty, trapezial excision with tissue interposition with or without ligament reconstruction, and total joint arthroplasty. A biodegradable T-shaped TMC device made of a degradable polycaprolactone-based polyurethaneurea (Artelon; Artimplant AB, Sweden) has been used in clinical pilot studies in Sweden [26]. The Artelon device serves two purposes: (1)to resurface the distal part of the trapezium and (2)to stabilize the TMC joint by augmentation of the joint capsule without subsequent shortening of the thumb that may cause decreased pinch strength [17, 36]. The complete hydrolysis of the spacer takes approximately six years [16]. When the hydrolysis is completed, part of the degraded material (approximately 50% of the initial weight) remains incorporated at the site of implantation [26].

Fifteen patients with radiographically verified, isolated stage 3 TMC osteoarthritis as described by Eaton and Glickel [13], were included in an open, controlled prospective study [26]. Five patients received the Artelon TMC Spacer anchored to bone with osteosutures, five patient were treated with tendon arthroplasty using the long abductor of the thumb (APL), and five patients received the Artelon TMC Spacer anchored with titanium screws. Implantation of the Artelon TMC Spacer was performed after removal of the distal 2 mm of the trapezium. A transient inflammatory reaction with moderate local swelling and tenderness at 2 weeks post-operatively that resolved without intervention, was noted in two patients who received the spacer. No other post-surgical complications were reported. Outcomes at three years were equivalent in terms of pain relief, ability to flatten the hand and range of motion among the three cohorts. The pinch strength measured by tripod pinch and key pinch (lateral pinch) was significantly higher in the spacer group compared with the APL group. Histologic specimens taken from one patient at 6 months (during removal of a titanium screw owing to discomfort) showed bone in contact with Artelon fibers without intervening structures as well as soft tissue in-growth into the woven structure at the periphery. There were no chronic inflammatory cells or any evidence of foreign-body response to the spacer. These initial results are promising and further clinical assessment of this device is ongoing.

Metacarpal/Phalangeal Injuries

Fracture Fixation

Treatment of metacarpal and phalangeal fractures requires a balance between providing mechanical stability to allow for early mobilization during post-operative rehabilitation while causing the least disruption to surrounding soft tissues. The deformity in metacarpal fractures is typically apex dorsal while proximal phalangeal fractures typically deform in an apex volar pattern due to the deforming effects of the extrinsic and intrinsic musculature of the hand. In fractures of either bone there are variable degrees of rotational or shortening forces depending on the specific fracture pattern [7]. Any form of fracture fixation must be sufficiently strong to counteract these forces.

Kirschner wire (K wire) fixation is considered by many to be a highly reproducible and useful method of operative treatment of fractures of tubular bones of the hand given the limited amount of soft tissue exposure required for placement. This treatment method is not without complications. Unless these are left protruding outside the skin, they require removal which may increase risk to soft tissues. On the other hand, when they are cut long to increase the ease of removal they can cause skin ulceration and be associated with pin tract infection. The inability to cut them flush to the bone may also interfere with free gliding of tendons inhibiting early range of motion rehabilitation protocols.

The use of bio-absorbable implants in the treatment of metacarpal and phalangeal fractures has many potential benefits. They do not require a later procedure for removal. They can be cut flush to the bone to decrease soft tissue irritation and may decrease the rate of infection as they do not leave the skin open to potential pin site infections. They are also radiolucent which aids in radiographic assessment of healing. While not in widespread use, initial studies are promising in that bio-absorbables may offer another treatment choice in the management of hand fractures.

In a cadaveric biomechanical study Fitoussi et al. (1998) compared the mechanical rigidity of K-wire to bio-absorbable pin fixation in proximal phalangeal fractures. Transverse and oblique osteotomy models were tested. Transverse fractures were treated with either two cross pins or one oblique pin with wire loop. Oblique fractures were treated with either two cross pins, two or three oblique pins. Metallic and bio-absorbable implants were found to be mechanically comparable under apex volar bending and compression forces. Bio-absorbable pins failed under torsional loads significantly earlier than the metal pins [14]. In a combined biomechanical and clinical study on extra-articular fractures in the hand 1.5 mm PGA rods (Biofix: Bioscience Ltd, Tampere Finland) were found to have 73% reduction in bending strength when implanted into bone and 64.4% reduction after implantation into subcutaneous tissue [22]. At three weeks all implants extracted were fragmented. The clinical trial consisted of 30 patients randomized to treatment either with 1.5mm or 2mm PGA rods or K-wire with wire loop added for further stability given the bio-absorbable implant was known to degrade to zero strength at three weeks. Patients were followed to 24 weeks and bony union was noted in all patients except one in the study group that became displaced at five weeks requiring re-operation attributed to faulty wiring technique and one patient in the control group that required re-operation for loss of reduction following K-wire migration. Both patients requiring re-operation went onto fracture healing by eight weeks. All patients except the two requiring re-operation returned to work ten to sixteen weeks after injury and no allergic reactions were noted in the study group.

With the development of self-reinforced bio-absorbable implants, the strength of fixation is increased and maintained for longer periods than the PGA pins tested in initial studies. The biomechanical results obtained with the use of non-reinforced bio-absorbable plates have also been less promising [10]. Bio-absorbable self-reinforced miniplates and screws have been developed for applications in craniomaxillofacial surgery and have recently been adapted for use in hand surgery.

Waris et al (2002) performed a biomechanical study using a pig metacarpal osteotomy model investigating the fixation stabilities of self-reinforced bioabsorbable SR-PLLA pins, and SR-P(L/DL)LA 70/30 screws and miniplates compared with those of standard metallic fixation. In this study, two interfragmentary 2.0 mm SR-P(L/DL)LA 70/30 screws provided similar fixation rigidity to two 1.5mm K-wires. SR-P(L/DL)LA 70/30 screws and 1.5mm SR-PLLA pins also showed similar rigidities in palmar and dorsal apex loading tests; however the screws were noted to have significantly increased rigidity when tested in lateral apex bending and in torsion. The SR-P(L/DL)LA screws did not show any statistically significant difference from titanium lag screws under bending or torsional stresses. The use of a single interfragmentary bio-absorbable screw provided low rotational rigidity as the bio-absorbable miniplate implant screws can not be applied as a lag screw barring interfragmentary compression. SR-P(L/DL)LA and titanium plating showed the highest mean values of failure torque and did not differ statistically from each other but the titanium plating had statistically significant greater rigidity [40].

While initial biochemical studies present data to suggest that newer self-reinforced bioabsorbable implants offer mechanical stability only slightly less than that of metallic implants [14, 23, 30, 38, 40] there are very few clinical studies available assessing the in-vivo behavior of these devices. In a case report of treatment with self-reinforced miniplates in complex hand injuries of three patients, all three patients went onto union without signs of plate failure [41]. There were no clinical signs of adverse reactions including sterile abscess formation, local irritation or swelling indicative of foreign body reactions to the implants. Arata et al (2003) reported a series of 26 cases of digital replantation using an intramedullary PLLA rod for the fixation of diaphyseal fractures. One case of transient bone resorption was observed but all patients went on to bony union and there were no reports of infection [3].

The ability to cut bio-absorbable implants directly at a bony surface presents an obvious potential benefit in the treatment of peri- or intra-articular fractures. Pelto-Vasenius et al. (1996) reported clinical results in the treatment of 13 metacarpal and phalangeal fractures, 12 of which were intra-articular using SR-PLLA and SR-PGA pins of 1.1, 1.5 and 2.0mm diameter. All fractures went on to bony union with report of only one minor re-displacement in a comminuted phalangeal fracture. Results of treatment specific to Bennett's fracture using similar methodology by the same surgeon were poor with only two of five patients having satisfactory results [29].

The treatment of hand fractures with bio-absorbable implants is still in its infancy, and as the experience of surgeons grows and industry follows with further development of devices, larger scale randomized controlled clinical studies are required to better understand the potential benefits and pitfalls of this new technology.

Soft Tissue Injury

The use of bio-absorbable suture anchors in the treatment of soft tissue injuries is commonly used in arthroscopic procedures of both the knee and shoulder. PLA/PGA composite anchors used in rotator cuff repairs have been shown to have comparable strength to metal anchors. Bio-absorbable suture anchors are used less frequently for soft tissue repairs in hand surgery. Their most notable use is in the repair of ulnar collateral ligaments of the thumb and repair of the scapholunate ligament. Vihtonen et al. reported excellent results in the treatment of 70 patients with total rupture of the ulnar collateral ligament of the first metacarpophalangeal joint of the thumb (skier's / gamekeeper's thumb) with SR-PLLA mini-tacks. Sixty-nine out of 70 patients healed without complication [44].

Complications

Immune Response

As bio-absorbable implants undergo degradation via hydrolysis, patients treated with PGA implants were noted to have foreign body reactions at a rate close to 5% [9]. Of 2528 patients treated with bio-absorbable pins, rods, bolts, and screws made of PGA or PLA from 1985-1995 at the University Hospital, Helsinki, 108 developed a clinically significant local inflammatory, sterile tissue reaction. The incidences were 5.3% (107 of 2037) with PGA implants and 0.2% (one of 491) with a PLA implant. This study excluded painless transient minor swelling which is also a frequently reported phenomenon [26, 33, 40]. The incidence varied among anatomic sites of implantation, from 1.8% in fractures of the radial head to 25% of scaphoid nonunions.

The overall volume of the implant did not affect the rate of incidence of soft tissue reaction; however the geometry of the implant did. Screws and serrated bolts had a statistically significant higher incidence of adverse tissue responses than pins and rods. In theory the larger surface area in contact with the host tissue increased the cellular reactivity and allowed for areas along the screw threads where an incubation process for an adverse tissue reaction could occur. Radiographs obtained at the time of presentation showed evidence of osteolysis along the implant tracks in 62 patients (57.4%). The implants manufactured between 1985 and 1988 included an additive green aromatic quinone dye within the polymer as a stain which increased the risk of a reaction ($p<0.001$) and was not included in implants produced after 1989. The rate of non-infectious foreign-body reaction after removal of the dye from the implants was 2.3% in PGA and 0% in PLA implants [34].

The many reports of foreign body reactions spurred study of the nature of the immune response to PGA implants. In aspirates performed from two patients following treatment of medial malleolar fractures with PGA Biofix implants the main cell type was a small lymphocyte with few monocytes [35]. In vitro investigation following this clinical observation, revealed that PGA-induced MHC locus II antigen and IL-2R activation marker expression was seen when peripheral blood mononuclear cells were cultured with supplemented PGA. This expression was greater than in negative controls but significantly less than that seen in PPD antigen driven lymphocyte response, suggesting that while PGA is an immunologically inert implant material, the slight non-specific lymphocyte activation is caused by induction of inflammatory mononuclear cell migration and adhesion to PGA implants.

Bacterial Infection

In the largest cohort reported, a review of 2,500 patients from the University of Helsinki managed using bio-absorbable devices, the overall bacterial infection rate was 3.6% [34]. This is similar to the rate reported for treatment with metallic implants.

Conclusions

While new technology is always on the horizon, it is the judicious implementation of this technology with vigilant preclinical and clinical study that allows surgical outcomes to improve. It must be understood that while bio-absorbable implants offer a multitude of potential benefits to problems experienced by hand surgeons world-wide, they are not free from their own individual complications.

References

[1] Akmaz, I; Kiral, A; Pehlivan, O; Mahirogullari, M; Solakoglu, C; Rodop, O. Biodegradable Implants in the Treatment of Scaphoid Nonunions. *Int Orthop.*, 2004, 25, 261-266.

[2] An, YH; Woolf, SK; Friedman, RJ. Pre-clinical in vivo evaluation of orthopaedic bioabsorbable devices. *Biomaterials.*, 2000, 21, 2635-2652.

[3] Arata, J; Ishikawa, K; Sawabe, K; Soeda, H; Kitayama, T. Osteosynthesis in digital replantation using bioabsorbable rods. *Annals of Plast. Surg.* 2003, 50, 350-353.

[4] Arora, RA; Lutz, M; Hennerbichler, A; Krappinger, D; Espen, D; Gabl, M. Complications Following Internal Fixation of Unstable Distal Radius Fractures and a Palmar Locking Plate. *J. Orthop. Trauma.*, 2007, 21, 5: 316-322

[5] Ashammakhi, N; Peltoniemi, H; Waris, E; Suuronen, R; Serlo, W; Kellomaki M; Törmälä, P; Waris, T. Developments in Craniomaxillofacial Surgery: Use of Self-

Reinforced Bioabsorbable Osteofixation Devices. *Plast. Recons. Surgery.*, 2001, 108, 167-180.

[6] Bergsma, JE, de Bruijn, WC, Rozema, FR, Bos, RR; Boering, G. Late Degradation Tissue Response to Poly (L-Lactide) Bone Plates and Screws. *Biomaterials.*, 1995, 16, 25-31.

[7] Black, D; Mann, R; Constin, R; Daniels, A. Comparison of internal fixation techniques in metacarpal fractures. *J. Hand Surg.*, 1982, 10A, 466-472.

[8] Böstman, O; Hirvensalo, E; Makinen, J; Rokkanen, P. Foreign Body Reactions to Fracture Fixation Implants of Biodegradable Synthetic Polymers. *J. Bone Joint. Surg.*, 1990, 72B, 592-596.

[9] Böstman, OM; Pihlajamaki, HK. Adverse Tissue Reactions to Bioabsorbable Fixation Devices. *Clin Orthop,* 2000, 371, 216-227.

[10] Bozic, KJ; Perez, LE; Wilson, DR; Fitzgibbons, PG; Jupiter, JB. Mechanical Testing of Bioresorbable Implants for Use in Metacarpal Fracture Fixation. *J. Hand Surg.*, 2001, 26A, 755-761.

[11] Campbell, DA. Open Reduction Internal Fixation of Intra-articular and Unstable Fractures of the Distal Radius Using the AO Distal Radius Plate. *J .Hand Surg.*, 2000, 25B, 528-534.

[12] Carter, PR; Frederick, HA; Laseter, GF. Open Reduction Internal Fixation of Unstable Distal Radius Fractures with a Low-Profile Plate: A Multicenter Study of 73 Fractures. *J. Hand Surg.*, 1998, 23A, 300-3007.

[13] Eaton, R; Glickel, S. Trapeziometacarpal osteoarthritis staging as a rationale for treatment. *Hand Clin.*, 1987, 3, 455-469.

[14] Fitoussi, F; Lu, W; Ip WY, Chow, SP. Mechanical Properties of Absorbable Implants in Finger Fractures. *J. Hand Surg* .1998, 23B, 1:79-83.

[15] Gangopadhyay, S; Ravi, K; Packer, G. Dorsal Plating of Unstable Distal Radius Fractures Using a Bioabsorbable Plating System and Bone Substitute. *J. Hand Surg.,* 2006, 31B, 1:93-100.

[16] Gisselfalt, K; Edberg, B; Flodin, P. Synthesis and properties of degradable poly (urethane urea) s to be used for ligament reconstructions. *Biomacromolecules.*, 2002, 3, 951-958.

[17] Hartigan, B; Stern, P; Kiefhaber, T. Thumb carpometacarpal osteoarthritis: arthrodesis compared with ligament reconstruction and tendon interposition. *J. Bone Joint Surg.,* 2001, 83A, 1470-1478.

[18] Howard, AC; Stanley, D; Getty, CJ. Wrist Arthrodesis in Rheumatoid Arthritis. A Comparison of Two Methods of Fusion. *J. Hand Surg.*, 1993, 18B, 377-380.

[19] Jakob, M; Rikli, DA; Regazzoni, D. Fracture of the Distal Radius Treated by Internal Fixation and Early Function. A Prospective Study of 73 Consecutive Patients. *J. Bone Joint Surg.*, 2000, 82B, 320-324.

[20] Juutilainen, T; Pätiälä, H. Arthrodesis in Rheumatoid Arthritis using Absorbable Screws and Rods. *Scand J. Rheumatol.*, 1995, 24, 228-233.

[21] Kujala, S; Raatikainene, T; Kaarela, O; Ashammakhi, N; Rynanen, J. Successful Treatment of Scaphoid Fractures and Nonunions Using Bioabsorbable Screws: Report of Six Cases. *J. Hand Surg.*, 2004, 29A, 68-73.

[22] Kumta, SM; Spinner, R; Leung, PC. Absorbable Intramedullary Implants for Hand Fractures: Animal Experiments and Clinical Trial. *J. Bone Joint. Surg.,* 1992, 74B, 563-566.

[23] Lionelli, GT; Korentager, RA. Biomechanical Failure of Metacarpal Fracture Resorbable Plate Fixation. *Ann. Plast Surg*., 2002, 49, 2:202-206.

[24] Majola, A; Vainiopaa, S; Vihtonen, K; Vasenius, J; Törmälä, P; Rokkanen, P. Intramedullary fixation of cortical bone osteotomies with self-reinforced polylactic rods in rabbits. *Int. Orthop*., 1992, 16, 1:101-108

[25] Mittal, R; Morley, J; Dinopoulos, H; Drakoulakis, E; Vermani, E; Giannoudi, P. Use of bio-resorbable implants for stablisation of distal radius fractures: the United Kingdom patients' perspective. *Injury.,* 2005, 36, 2:333-338

[26] Nilsson, A; Liljensten, E; Bergstrom, C; Sollerman, C. Results From a Degradable TMC Joint Spacer (Artelon) Compared with Tendon Arthroplasty. *J. Hand Surg.,* 2005, 30A, 2:380-389.

[27] Pech, J; Sosna, A; Rybka, V; Pokorny, D. Wrist Arthrodesis in Rheumatoid Arthritis. A New Technique Using Internal Fixation. *J .Hand Surg*., 1998, 78B, 783-786.

[28] Pelto-Vasenius, K; Hirvensalo, E; Böstman, O; Rokkanen, P. Fixation of scaphoid delayed union and nonunion with absorbable polyglycolide pin of Herbert screw. Consolidation and functional results. *Arch. Orthop. Trauma Surg*., 1995, 114, 347-351

[29] Pelto-Vasenius, K; Hirvensalo, E; Rokkanen, P. Absorbable pins in the treatment on hand fractures. *Ann. Chir. Gynacol*., 1996, 85, 4:353-358.

[30] Pihlajamaki, H; Böstman, O; Hirvensalo, E; Törmälä, P; Rokkanen, P. Absorbable Pins of Self-Reinforced Poly-L-Lactic Acid for Fixation of Fractures and Osteotomies. *J. Bone Joint Surg*., 1992, 74B, 563-566.

[31] Rehak, D; Kasper, P; Baratz, M; Hagberg, WC; McClaine, E; Imbriglia, JE. A Comparison of Plate and Pin Fixation for Arthrodesis of the Rheumatoid Wrist. *Orthopedics*., 2000, 23, 43-48.

[32] Ring, D; Jupiter, J; Brennwald, J; Buchler, U; Hastings, H. 2nd. Prosective Multicenter Trial of a Plate for Dorsal Fixation of Distal Radius Fractures. *J. Hand Surg*., 1997, 22A, 777-784.

[33] Rokkanen, P; Böstman, O; Hirvensalo, E; Makela, E; Partio, E; Pätiälä, H; Vainionpaa, S; Vihtonen, K; Törmälä, P. Bioabsorbable Fixation in Orthopaedic Surgery and Traumatology. *Biomaterials,* 2000, 21, 2607-2613.

[34] Rokkanen, P; Böstman, O; Vainionpaa, S; Makela, A; Hirvensalo, E; Pario, E; Vihtonen, K; Pätiälä, H; Törmälä, P. Absorbable devices in fixation of fractures. *J. Trauma,* 1996, 40, 3S: 123-127.

[35] Santavirta, S; Konttinen, Y; Saito, T; Gronblad, M; Partio, E; Kemppinen P; Rokkanen P. Immune Response to Polyglycolic Acid Implants. *J. Bone Joint Surg. [Br],* 1990, 72, 597-600.

[36] Tomaino, M; Pellgrini, V; Jr, Burton, R. Arthroplasty of the basal joint of the thumb. Long-term follow-up after ligament reconstruction with tendon interposition. *J. Bone Joint Surg* .1995, 77A, 345-355.

[37] Törmälä, P. Biodegradable Self-Reinforced Composite Materials; Manufacturing Structure and Mechanical Properties. *Clin. Mater*., 1992, 10, 29-34.

[38] Waris, E; Ashammakhi, N; Happonen, H; Raatikainen, T; Kaarela, O; Törmälä, P; Santavirta, S; Konttinen, Y. Bioabsorbable miniplating versus metallic fixation of metacarpal fractures. *Clin. Orthop.Res.*, 2003, 410, 310-319.

[39] Waris, E; Ashammakhi, N; Kaarela, O; Raatikainen, T; Vasenius, J. Use of Bioabsorbable Osteofixation Devices in the Hand. *J. Hand Surg.*, 2004, 29B, 6:590-598.

[40] Waris, E; Ashmmakhi, N; Raatikainen, T; Tormala, P; Santavirta, S; Konttinene, YT. Self-Reinforced Bioabsorbable Versus Metallic Fixation Systems for Metacarpal and Phalangeal Fractures: A Biomechanical Study. *J. Hand Surg.*, 2002, 27A, 5:902-909.

[41] Waris, E; Harpf, C; Ninkovic, M; Ashammakhi, N. Self-Reinforced Bioabsorbable Miniplates for Skeletal Fixation in Complex Hand Injury: Three Case Reports. *J. Hand Surg.*, 2004, 29A, 3:452-457.

[42] Williams, D. Some observations on the role of cellular enzymes in the in-vivo degradation of polymers. *Corrosion and degradation of implant materials, American Society for Testing and Materials*, 1979, 61-75.

[43] Vasenius, J; Vainionpaa, S; Vihtonen, K; Makela, A; Rokkanen, P; Mero, M; Romala P. Comparison of In Vitro Hydrolysis, Subcutaneous and Intramedullary Implantation to Evaluate the Strength Retention of Absorbable Osteosynthesis Implants. *Biomaterials.*, 1990, 11, 501-504.

[44] Vihtonen, K; Juutilainen, T; Pätiälä, H; Rokkanen, P; Törmälä, P. Reinsertion of the ruptured ulnar collateral ligament of the metacarpophalangeal joint with an absorbable self-reinforced polylactide tack. *J. Hand Surg.*, 1993, 18B, 200-3.

[45] Voutilainen, N; Juutilainen, T; Pätiälä, H; Rokkenen, P. Arthodesis of the Wrist with Bioabsorbable Fixation in Patients with Rheumatoid Arthritis. *J. Hand Surg.*, 2002, 27B, 6:563-567.

[46] Voutilainen, N; Pätiälä, H; Juutilainen, T; Rokkanen, P. Long Term Results of Wrist Arthrodeses Fixed with Self-Reinforced Polylevolactic Acid Implants in Patients with Rheumatoid Arthritis. *Scand J. Rheumatol.*, 2001, 30, 3: 1149-153.

[47] Yamamuro, T; Matsusue, Y; Urchida, A; Shimada, K; Shimozaki, E; Kitaoka, K. Bioabsorbable Osteosynthetic Implants of Ultra High Strength Poly-L-Lactide. A Clinical Study. *Int. Orthop.*, 1994, 18, 332-340.

Index

B

C

D

E

F

G

H

I

N

Q

R

S

T

U

V

W

X